Preface

In the past hundred years, medicine has tried to acquire a scientific basis. Age-old prejudices and pointless procedures have been discarded in controlled study after study. Today, we take it for granted that the practice of medicine is evidence-based.

Yet in psychiatry the penetration of science has been imperfect. The discipline has swung wildly from fashion to fashion—from asylum care to psychoanalysis to lobotomy to psychopharmacology—without having an underlying scientific rationale for doing so. More than any other medical field, psychiatry has been guided by cultural preferences and political persuasions. We vaguely dislike the notion of "locking up" people or of shooting volts of electricity through their brains; we have a natural enlightened tropism toward psychotherapy and the enhancement of human reason and against the madness of unreason. None of these prejudices and preferences is in itself reprehensible, and all flow from a praiseworthy humanism. But prejudices and beliefs are not science. In a great disjunction, science and psychiatry have passed each other like two ships in the night.

Yet psychiatry cries out for science. To be sure, we can gauge the neurochemistry of the brain and assess its structures with the devices of neuroimaging. But the questions of clinical psychiatry are more complex than fluctuations in neurotransmitters or glucose uptake in the basal ganglia, where the brain gives up few of its secrets. Is there no other way to gain a window to the brain and gauge its activity in psychiatric illness? Yes, there is. Another system, the endocrine system, sets the biological rhythms of brain and body. Psychiatry was once fascinated with the endocrine system. Today, the adrenal and pituitary glands, and the hypothalamus within the brain, have lost their charm and arouse little interest.

Simultaneously, psychiatry also said adieu to another familiar historical concept, melancholia, as a diagnosis of severe depression. After the introduction of a new system of disease classification in 1980, the diagnosis of "major depression"—a heterogeneous assortment of varied illness entities and unhappiness states—swept the field. This is very interesting: At the same time that psychiatric interest in neurotransmitters such as serotonin quickened, the discipline embraced such new illnesses as "major depression" and "bipolar disorder." In understanding the seat of illness, there was a shift from the endocrine periphery to the neurotransmitter central, and in classification, there was a shift from such sturdy historical concepts as "melancholia" to the more faddish notions of "major depression" and "bipolar disorder." These two shifts are related. In both, the profession of psychiatry walked away from solid, well-verified knowledge into a botanical maze of fashion, commerce, and politics.

Melancholia is a serious illness. It involves the slowing of thought and mood, the absence of joy or pleasure in life, and profound changes in the body's daily rhythms. Max Fink and Michael Alan Taylor have defined it as "a recurrent, debilitating, pervasive brain disorder that alters mood, motor functions, thinking, cognition, perception and many basic physiological processes."[1] This book makes the point that melancholia has a biology of its own that is heavily entwined with the endocrine system. In coming to grips with the riddle of melancholia, psychiatry has this endocrine knowledge to draw upon, yet seldom does. This is a failure of science and of clinical practice.

How did this failure happen? Endocrine thinking in psychiatry rode a wave of great excitement in the 1970s and 1980s, and then it seeped away. Few clinicians today are curious about cortisol or thyroid-releasing hormone, two hormones with intimate relationships to behavior. While physicians might include assays of thyroid hormones when requesting laboratory tests, they are often incurious about the results unless a blood measure is wildly out of balance. As for the complex interrelationships among hypothalamus, pituitary, adrenal gland, and the rest of it, that material is learned once during medical school and rarely considered again thereafter.

There is a price to be paid for this endocrine distaste, just as there is a price for the profession's reluctance to contemplate convulsive

Endocrine Psychiatry

Endocrine Psychiatry

Solving the Riddle of Melancholia

Edward Shorter, PhD

Jason A. Hannah Professor of the History of Medicine
Professor of Psychiatry
Faculty of Medicine, University of Toronto
Toronto, Ontario, Canada

Max Fink, MD

Professor of Psychiatry and Neurology Emeritus
Stony Brook University School of Medicine
Stony Brook, New York

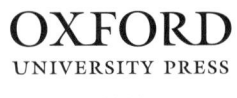

OXFORD
UNIVERSITY PRESS

2010

OXFORD

UNIVERSITY PRESS

Oxford University Press, Inc., publishes works that further
Oxford University's objective of excellence
in research, scholarship, and education.

Oxford   New York

Auckland   Cape Town   Dar es Salaam   Hong Kong   Karachi
Kuala Lumpur   Madrid   Melbourne   Mexico City   Nairobi
New Delhi   Shanghai   Taipei   Toronto

With offices in

Argentina   Austria   Brazil   Chile   Czech Republic   France   Greece
Guatemala   Hungary   Italy   Japan   Poland   Portugal   Singapore
South Korea   Switzerland   Thailand   Turkey   Ukraine   Vietnam

Published by Oxford University Press, Inc.
198 Madison Avenue, New York, New York 10016

www.oup.com

Oxford is a registered trademark of Oxford University Press

Library of Congress Cataloging-in-Publication Data

Shorter, Edward.
Endocrine psychiatry : solving the riddle of melancholia / by Edward Shorter, Max Fink.
p. ; cm.
Includes bibliographical references and index.
ISBN 978-0-19-973746-8
1. Depression, Mental—Endocrine aspects—Research—History.   I. Fink, Max, 1923–   II. Title.
[DNLM: 1. Depressive Disorder—history.   2. Depressive Disorder—complications.   3. Endocrine System
Diseases—complications.   4. History, 19th Century.   5. History, 20th Century.   6. History, 21st Century.
7. Neuroendocrinology—history.   8. Psychophysiology—history.   WM 11.1 S559e 2010]
RC537.S386 2010
616.85′27075—dc22
2009031261

1   3   5   7   9   8   6   4   2

Printed in the United States of America
on acid-free paper

Dedicated to the memory of Edward Sachar, who brought the neuroendocrines to the attention of clinical psychiatry; and to Bernard (Barney) Carroll, who dedicated his professional life to validating hypercortisolemia in the pathophysiology of severe depressive mood disorders.

therapy.[2] Melancholic illness, among the most serious of all psychiatric disorders, remains often imperfectly diagnosed and inadequately treated. We try to deliver the best possible care of patients, yet patient care suffers when important guides to understanding illness and meliorating symptoms are left fallow.

This endocrine indifference is typical of a wider pattern. A trail of discarded therapies and paradigms litters the history of psychiatry. Some, such as lobotomy and pouring cold water on women with "hysteria," will probably not again see the light of day. Others, such as electroconvulsive treatment and using the brain's electrical rhythms to study drug effects, have been prematurely cast aside—and urgently deserve a rebirth. Our interest today is on neurotransmitter levels and multicolor images of neuron–neuron interaction, on serotonin and dopamine, but cortisol may well offer a better marker of patients' woes than the principal neurotransmitters. This loss is particularly serious if the patients are melancholic. In mood disorders, there are important markers that have unjustly fallen into desuetude.

The rationale of this book is to urge a rebirth of endocrine approaches as a way of coming to grips with melancholia.

Endocrine psychiatry deserves a second look.

Acknowledgments

For financial support of this research, we are most grateful to the Scion Natural Science Association, Inc., the Canadian Institutes of Health Research (CIHR), and the Social Sciences and Humanities Research Council of Canada (SSHRC). We undertook archival research in several collections: notably, the Department of Special Collections, University of California-Irvine Libraries (Ralph W. Gerard papers); Brandeis University Archives (Sachar Collection); Eskind Biomedical Library, Vanderbilt University (International Neuropharmacology Archives, Carroll papers); and the archives of the American Psychiatric Association in Arlington, Virginia. Among individuals who permitted themselves to be interviewed were George Arana, Gregory Asnis, Ross Baldessarini, Walter Brown, Bernard (Barney) Carroll, Paula Clayton, Alexander (Sandy) Glassman, Uriel Halbreich, Donald F. Klein, Paul McHugh, Charles Nemeroff, Robert Rubin, David Rubinow, David Sachar, Raymond Sackler, Robert Spitzer, and Marvin Stein.

We are grateful to Walter Brown, Bernard Carroll, and Michael Alan Taylor for critically reading an earlier draft.

The paths of the researchers were greatly smoothed by the assistance of Heather Dichter, Jonathan Ruelens, and Ellen Tulchinsky. Susan Bélanger, research coordinator and administrator of the History of Medicine Program at the University of Toronto, has been a pearl beyond price.

Edward Shorter
Max Fink

Contents

Endocrine Psychiatry

1

Introduction

Why an interest in endocrine psychiatry? The history of endocrine psychiatry—or, to use its technical name, psychoneuroendocrinology—is a MEGO-style subject: "my eyes glaze over." Neuroendocrine approaches have largely vanished from consideration in clinical practice and even from research psychiatry. Endocrinology remains an arcane subspecialty of internal medicine, whose practitioners are more interested in the endocrine aspects of the organs of reproduction than in thyroid and adrenal glands. Yet the subject is important for medical practitioners because it may hold the key to stress-related abnormalities of behavior, particularly melancholia.

It was via an interest in the therapeutics of melancholic illness that we came to endocrine psychiatry. One of us, Max Fink, had spent many years encouraging greater use of electroconvulsive therapy (ECT), the effective treatment for melancholia. Both of us have a long-standing interest in melancholia as a life-threatening illness that possesses the paradoxical quality of responding dramatically to treatment. And Edward Shorter had recently published a history of electroconvulsive therapy, just as endocrine psychiatry flashed on our screen. It flashed because we became interested in a diagnostic test for melancholia, the dexamethasone suppression test (DST), which enjoyed a shot-put–like rise and fall: becoming fashionable (for good reasons) in the 1970s and 1980s, then plummeting to extinction. But the DST was a serviceable guide to melancholia and to gauging its prognosis: Why the baffling loss of interest in one of the few biological markers that psychiatry has discovered?

Thus we came to endocrine psychiatry, the oldest of the biological approaches to psychiatric illness, a subject deemed too obscure and marginal for anyone today save the dedicated endocrinologists buried in the medicine wards of hospitals.

Melancholia is a riddle. Patients commonly come with characteristic and easily identified symptoms—pathological slowing of thought and muscle, an almost psychotic image of self-unworth, crushing tiredness, and despair and pains so severe as to turn their thoughts to suicide. They also have a distinctive biological abnormality. They produce excesses of the hormone cortisol and have distinctive thyroid and sleep abnormalities. But the findings about cortisol and thyroid in particular give the disease a biological homogeneity that other psychiatric illnesses lack. Psychiatry has identified no distinctive physical findings in schizophrenia, anxiety, or non-melancholic depression. Seeing melancholia as a disease with as much of a biological root as mumps opens the prospect of learning its pathophysiology—its physical causes. Understanding the genesis of melancholia makes possible a better cure for it than electroconvulsive treatment, which, although highly effective, frightens many patients.

Solving the riddle of melancholia holds great promise. Understanding its roots in endocrines is a way station on a royal road, that same road that half a century ago led to antibiotics to solve the riddle of bacterial illness and to insulin to solve the riddle of diabetes. Endocrine psychiatry has a certitude of promise that warrants this journey.

There's a second reason for this writing, too, one that sees psychiatrists as physicians. The endocrine glands direct the attention of psychiatry to the entire body, not just to the regions above the neck. The entire body once figured prominently in the understanding of mental afflictions; today that image is out of style, and unconscious conflicts and neurotransmitters are accorded pride of place. Yet, psychiatrists are trained as physicians, and in their medical rotations as students and interns, they wear stethoscopes slung about their white jackets just as other physicians do. Suffering psychiatric patients certainly believe the entire body is involved, as they experience the aches and pains of depressive illness. Yet their therapists will probably limit the search for biological causes to the standard panel of blood and urine tests, if that.

The search for biological markers of mental disease has been ill served. Biological markers of diseases of the mind and brain are largely ignored in psychiatry, compared with the biochemical markers identifying cardiac damage or the abnormal electroencephalogram (EEG) in diagnosing epilepsy. Psychiatric illnesses are delineated by checking off symptoms, a process called "phenomenology." The presence of abnormal mood, peculiar thoughts, and abnormal vegetative signs defines a psychiatric disorder, according to a checklist in a diagnostic manual called the *DSM*, or *Diagnostic and Statistical Manual* of the American Psychiatric Association (APA). The manual identifies more than 300 different clusters of symptoms, each labeled as a psychiatric disorder with a checklist of its own. (This approach is slightingly referred to as "Chinese-menu psychiatry.") Such clustering is unsatisfactory because the symptoms are not specific or well defined; many overlap in different diagnoses, fluctuate in every patient, vary in severity and duration, and make a reliable biologically based diagnosis almost impossible.

Today's psychiatry does have some useful biological markers. Fever points to a toxic or infectious process; a positive serological test points to an infection with syphilis; an abnormal EEG is a marker of a seizure disorder; the response to lorazepam is a marker for catatonia; the response to a carbon dioxide challenge is a marker for panic disorder; and abnormal thyroid function points to a metabolic error. A certain EEG pattern helps diagnose the kind of hyperactivity in children that responds to stimulant treatment.[1] As the following pages make clear, an abnormal level of the hormone cortisol and an inadequate reaction to dexamethasone, an artificial steroid, are markers of melancholia.

These few biological markers leave much abnormal behavior without biological roots. The authors consider it urgent to drag psychiatry closer to medicine, to trim it closer to the "medical model," with less consideration of the "biopsychosocial model," a concept that focuses interest on the patient's personal life and social setting rather than on brain and systemic biology.

It is an accepted tenet that effective psychiatrists should be attentive to the patient, his illness, personal history, and social universe. But few clinicians are curious about the subject's endocrine system, about the hypothalamus and adrenal glands, because they have not been trained to see the importance of these organs in behavior. Their incuriosity is quite comparable to an incuriosity about electroconvulsive therapy, a treatment that has followed a similar trajectory: looming into prominence at its origin, rejected and cast aside, and recently resurrected. On other occasions we have described this curious history.[2] Endocrine psychiatry offers an interesting counterpart: a period of intense interest and a rapid rise and fall after the 1970s, without the parallel benefit of resurgence that ECT enjoys today. We rummage about in the treasury book of psychiatry's past, find these little nuggets, and brandish them as ripe for rediscovery.

Psychiatrists' lack of interest today in their endocrine past has been matched by that of historians. With few exceptions, the historians of medicine have shied away from the subject as if it were distant from humanistic learning and Freudian triumphs.[3] The history of the secretions of the adrenal gland! Oh dear, no.

How does one nudge psychiatry closer to medicine? For one thing, clinical medicine is interested in disease markers and biological tests. Psychiatry lacks both, as it relies on what the patient says to make the diagnosis. One cannot imagine a cardiologist's limiting diagnostic considerations to the patient's account of chest pain or a neurologist's offering a diagnosis of headache based on the description of the headache alone.

The lack of tests is not an inherent limitation in the nature of psychiatric knowledge about which we wring our hands in vain. There are means of roughly assessing what is going on in the brain and body to produce disordered behavior. Yet the official manual of diagnosis, the *Diagnostic and Statistical Manual* series of the APA, explicitly rejects any biological test to verify a diagnosis made by symptom check-off. When *DSM-III*, the beginning of the new *DSM* series, was drafted in 1980, the disease designers explicitly decided that biological measures were unhelpful. The chairman, Robert Spitzer, and the members of the *DSM* Task Force rejected tests that might demarcate patients within a psychiatric class, such as measures of cortisol in order to chisel out melancholia from the vague class of "mood disorders."[4] In a later interview, Task Force member Paula Clayton was asked by the authors: "Why were laboratory tests discarded?"

Clayton replied, "There was no way to make sure that a test really applied to a disease."[5]

But endocrine medicine does offer tests and markers. In addition to the endocrine system, the immune system, electrophysiology, and the response to specific challenges such as benzodiazepines in catatonia: all provide markers of clinical value. If one views psychiatric illness as a disorder of the body rather than of just the brain and mind, physical markers spring forth, much like pulses that are found all over the body and not just at the radial artery of the wrist. The mindset of the *DSM* classification has constricted our gaze, causing the low levels of treatment success and the high incidence of "treatment resistance" seen in today's clinical practice. Both derive from the constricted visual field of *DSM* thinking.

This book is about much more than biological markers, but, right up front, the markers that interest us are abnormalities of the secretions of the hypothalamus, the pituitary, the thyroid, and the adrenal glands. Their abnormalities form a fundamental part of clinical psychiatry. Two chapters of the book are devoted to a biological marker that older clinicians may well have forgotten and younger ones have never heard of: the dexamethasone suppression test. The test was conceived in the late 1960s as specific for melancholia; it soared in popularity in the misunderstood belief that it represented a screening test for "depression," then collapsed in collective disappointment as the *DSM-III* definition of depression turned out to be so non-specific as to defy any test. Apropos this error, one of us (Fink) wrote: "Rejection [of the DST] for a quarter of a century and the profession's failure to devise any more reliable measure has left psychiatric diagnosis of mood disorders in a shambles.... Neuroendocrine tests define a characteristic population of depressed patients best labeled 'melancholic.'"[6] The DST tugged psychiatry in the direction of the brain and body as a platform for the mind.

But the brain and body have always been something of a no-go zone for practicing psychiatrists. Joel Elkes, a founder of modern biological psychiatry, talked about his early days in Birmingham, England, during the Second World War.

> No Beckmann [spectrophotometer], no fluid fraction collector, no radioimmunoassay in those days. So, you get the chilled brain, sit down patiently and dissect it into thirteen regional samples, blowing on your freezing fingers as you go along.... "Elkes," a senior colleague tells me, "don't be a fool. Work on the heart, work on the gut, but get out of the brain. The brain is a sticky mess, and you'll come to a sticky end."[7]

Indeed, in those days the difference was that the heart and the gut could be examined, but the brain, practically speaking, could not. Portuguese neurologist Egas Moniz introduced cerebral angiography in 1927, but for most psychiatric purposes the procedure was uninformative. Neuropathology, studied with a microscope, had been practiced for a century before and was useful in defining the pathology of inherited neuron metabolic disorders, such as Tay-Sachs-Schaffer syndrome, a pediatric metabolic disorder resulting in early death.[8] Yet the practical results for clinical psychiatry could be counted on the fingers of the hand. When Joel Elkes began research in the 1940s, there was, aside from a study of the cerebrospinal fluid, simply no way to see into the brain and determine what was happening to its chemistry.

An obvious tactic was to probe the brain chemically and observe the results in the changed behavior of patients, or at least in changes in physiological and chemical measures. Since the work of Geoffrey Harris in 1948, it has been clear that the pituitary gland was directed by higher structures in the brain. Poking at the endocrine system chemically and observing the results might bring light to the darkness that enveloped the contents of the cranium. It offered a way to explore the ill brain. "In major depressive illness, the neuroendocrine system serves as a window into the brain", as Charles Nemeroff and colleagues once pointed out.[9]

Yet the profession of psychiatry marginalized the study of the endocrine system. Clinicians tutored in psychoanalysis and psychotherapy found its wet complexity daunting compared with the comfortable humanism of the interview with its reports of dreams. The rush toward neurotransmitters in the 1960s elbowed aside aspects of research that were less profitable for the pharmaceutical industry. Thus, aside from a brief strut upon central stage in the 1970s and 1980s, endocrine psychiatry has been a stepchild.

This was a mistake.

Three body systems are relevant to biological psychiatry. One encompasses the glandular products that pass into the bloodstream from "the organs of internal secretion." Within the bloodstream, they have broad effects on all the cells of the body.

A second system is that of the *neurohumors*, or the chemical messengers that carry stimulating or inhibiting signals between the nerve cells. Strictly speaking, neurohumors are also found in the nervous tissues all over the body, between the nerve cells in the heart, gut, or bladder. In the nervous system, these chemicals are restricted to the limited spaces, or synapses, between brain cells. Today, they are called *neurotransmitters*, and the bulk of research in psychiatry is focused on them rather than the endocrines.

The third system is the *immune system*, defined as the science of neuropsychoimmunology. (The immune system is the tissue-defense response to a foreign protein, as from a pathogen or malignant cell. The response is marked by the release of cytokines and other chemicals that destroy the pathogen.) The immune reactions in the brain and body are diverse. The science of neuropsychoimmunology has a small following, drowned out by the bellowing about "deficient serotonin" and SSRI-style inhibitors of its reuptake, such as Prozac.

Over the years, two research approaches have been applied to endocrinology—ablation of glands to reduce secretions or stimulation to increase their outflow. Somatic diseases of the body are associated with glandular excess (hyperthyroidism) and glandular deficiency (diabetes, hypothyroidism). The question in psychiatric disorders is: With what glandular excesses and deficiencies are diseases of the brain and mind associated? We are more likely to find answers if we study the problems rather than ignore them. This book is a history, pointing to the past, hopefully as prologue.

Our questions have been long in brewing. As Richard Michael and James Gibbons at the Institute of Psychiatry of the Maudsley Hospital in London pointed out in 1963, on the threshold of the new endocrine psychiatry, "For the past 70 years psychiatrists have treasured the illusion that the solution of several etiological problems in psychiatry only awaited advances in the endocrinological field." They pointed out that Emil Kraepelin, the founder of the modern classification of psychiatric disease, had once considered dementia praecox an endocrine disorder and that Sigmund Freud anticipated the advent of hormone treatments for some conditions. "A whole series of speculative treatments has at one time or another been attempted with every variety of endocrine preparation. The inevitable failure of such methods caused endocrinological psychiatry . . . to fall into disrepute."[10]

Then in the late 1950s, a revival of endocrine thinking occurred with the discovery of the link between high serum cortisol levels and illness. This link stimulated forty years of fast-lane science, using the new investigative technique of radioimmune assay, a test that uses radiolabeling to detect the concentration of any substance capable of evoking a specific antibody response. In an outpouring of research of great relevance to endocrinology, there have been only a few clinically relevant findings for psychiatrists. Yet they are important ones.

In depressive mood disorders, the endocrine link from hypothalamus in the brain, via the pituitary gland, to the adrenal glands—called the HPA axis—is activated. The process starts in the brain: most immediately in the hypothalamus, the region sitting at the base of the brain. Oversecretion continues at every level in the HPA axis, from adrenocorticotrophic hormone (ACTH) in the pituitary to cortisol in the adrenal gland. (Abnormalities of the HPA axis may be measured, among other procedures, by variations in serum levels of cortisol and the DST.) On the thyroid side, patients may have a blunted, or deadened, pituitary response to the thyroid releasing factor secreted by the hypothalamus. (Terms: for thyroid, the hormone secreted by the pituitary is called thyroid-stimulating hormone [TSH]. On the adrenal side, the pituitary secretes ACTH in response to corticotropin-releasing hormone [CRH], also called corticotropin-releasing factor [CRF], secreted by the hypothalamus. Thyrotropin-releasing hormone [TRH] is often called thyrotropin-releasing factor [TRF]; the expressions "hormone" and "factor" are used interchangeably in the literature.) Moreover, abnormalities are often simultaneously present in the same patients.

But let's not get too far into findings, as we're just at the beginning of the story. Let's go for the big picture: the brain–body relationship. The past hundred years have seen an ongoing struggle within psychiatry about how to conceive this relationship. There have been three camps: mind, brain, and brain and body.

For many years, proponents of the mind were in ascendance. Psychoanalysis, which dominated psychiatry in the middle third of the twentieth century, dealt only with the mind and the presumed struggle among its conscious and unconscious layers, the known recollections in awareness and those hidden by protecting energies.

The biological approach to psychiatry that surged into fashion after the 1970s privileged mainly the brain and displayed an overwhelming interest in neurotransmitters, neuroimaging, and neurogenetics. What the adrenals, thyroid, and autonomic nervous system were doing mattered little to this biological psychiatry.

The brain-and-body approach has decidedly been an underdog, yet it has blossomed from time to time, seeing psychiatric events as manifestations of vast physiological currents that sweep across the entire body. This interpretation goes back to the very beginning of psychiatry as a discipline late in the eighteenth century, when clinicians were still in the grip of the doctrine of the "humors," fluids that were presumed to circulate in the body and affect the tissues. Black bile, for example, was thought to be the humor that caused melancholia. Black bile in the body affected the brain, an essentially physiological proposition. Vincenzo Chiarugi, professor of psychiatry in Florence, Italy, and among the founders of the discipline, described in 1794 a herdsman of about forty years of age who was brought to the psychiatric hospital: "As a result of strong emotional conflicts, he became melancholic, and following a copious bleeding, in a very short time he became manic." It was germane for Chiarugi that "his liver and spleen were noticeably obstructed; hence, he was repeatedly purged with cream of tartar." Over the following months, the patient's mania abated. "However, on the three occasions that he lost his appetite, he was made to vomit with an appropriate dose of tartar emetic; consequently, abundant relief from bilious matter was obtained." "In the following September, having been greatly helped by about twenty general tepid baths, he was able to go home completely cured, even of the obstructions in his lower abdomen."[11] For psychiatrists of Chiarugi's generation, the tides of the body were intimately linked to the passions of the spirit; once rid of the "bilious matter" in the stomach, the patient was restored to psychic health.

By the time of English psychiatrist Henry Maudsley, physician to the West London Hospital in the 1860s, a proper "physiological psychiatry," divorced from the now-discredited humors, had established itself. Maudsley told readers in his 1867 textbook *The Physiology and Pathology of the Mind*, "I have had in view throughout this work . . . to treat of mental phenomena from a physiological rather than from a metaphysical point of view." (This was a reference to previous psychiatrists' fixation upon "moral"—meaning religious and social—causes of insanity.) Maudsley implicated an inheritable degeneration of the nervous system affecting the entire body:

An innate taint or infirmity of nervous element may modify in a striking manner the mode of manifestation of other diseases; where it exists, gout flying about the body may produce obscure nervous symptoms, so as greatly to puzzle the inexperienced practitioner, and the syphilitic poison is similarly apt to seize upon the weak part, and to give rise to severe nervous symptoms . . . . A prenatal disease which does not specially affect the nervous system may . . . be at the foundation of a delicate nervous constitution in the offspring: phthisis [tuberculosis], scrofula [cervical lymph node tuberculosis], syphilis, perhaps also gout and diabetes, may act thus banefully.[12]

For Maudsley, the practice of psychiatry was part of internal medicine and neurology.

The familiar distinction between reactive and endogenous depression goes back to members of the German school of psychopathology in the early twentieth century: endogenous depression affected the entire body; reactive, solely the mental layer of emotions. It was Kurt Schneider, professor of psychiatry in Cologne and author of the "Schneiderian criteria" of schizophrenia, who distinguished "endogenous depression" and "reactive depression" in 1920.[13] Endogenous depression, he said, represented a disturbance of the body's "vital" feelings, which were found in the physical plane of life itself. Schneider described this vital feeling as follows: "[It] participates in the body's entire sense of the sum of its functions [*Gesamtausdehnungscharakter des Leibes*], without being localized in any particular part." "In such a feeling we grasp life itself, and in this feeling something is imparted to us: ascent, decline, health, illness, [and] danger." Endogenous depressions, Schneider believed, came on spontaneously and were "unprovoked", meaning not triggered by stress; they were a bubble on the foam of the body's physiological ebbs and floods.

Today as well, many patients with severe depression report having Schneider's "entire feeling" of their body affected. When in 2004 Colleen Kelly, a depression sufferer, testified to an advisory committee of the Food and Drug Administration (FDA), she said, "Our illness is embedded in our physical bodies, ourselves. We are prisoners there."[14] Severe depression is a disorder (or dysfunction) of the whole body.

Reactive depression, by contrast, was for Schneider a disorder of the affective plane (*seelische Gefühle*), caused by social and family problems and expressed in sadness. Reactive depressions did not necessarily include what came to be called "neurovegetative" or "autonomic" symptoms touching the entire body. For Schneider, the difference between "reactive" and "vital" (endogenous) was their insertion at different "emotional layers."

The Schneiderian distinction between "reactive" and "endogenous" gradually drifted out of focus over the years; *reactive* came to mean a response to bad news, *endogenous* to mean a spontaneous disorder, not moved by external events. This German tradition of psychopathology sheet-anchored the practice of seeing symptoms as the result of physiological events sweeping across the entire body, not just as a result of psychological dysphoria or unconscious conflict.

Endocrine psychiatrists are the descendants of the psychiatric tradition of physiological psychiatry, beginning with the Ancients and progressing to the organic psychiatrists of the nineteenth century and the psychopathologists of the early twentieth. Standing at the intersection of the body's three great signaling systems—the endocrine, nervous, and immune—endocrine psychiatrists are exquisitely attuned to psychiatric illness as borne by the tides of cortisol, the pituitary and hypothalamic hormones, and even the gonadotropins that rush back and forth across the circulation of the entire body and brain. Joel Elkes evoked events at this intersection: "The three great information systems in the body-mind, the endocrine, nervous, and immune system, use common elements in the languages they share. In the society of cells within the skin, chemical signals travel swiftly from one system to the other. We are at the earliest beginnings of understanding this compact, confusing and puzzling traffic."

Elkes noted that our understanding of infectious illness has made great gains by pinning down the specific actions in the body of pathogens and their therapeutics. But psychiatry was different. "The disorders we are called on to treat are unlikely to be focal disorders [localized lesions]. More likely, they may turn out to be disorders of molecular communication in an informational network that includes the brain in an ancient partnership with the nervous and endocrine system. Molecular signals of close affinity travel ceaselessly both ways." So, for psychiatry, no single lesions, no "magic bullets," as German bacteriologist Paul Ehrlich once conceived the specificity of pharmacological action.[15] Elkes contended, "It is the cascade, the statistical chatter and conversation in chemically 'labeled' nets that may give us a glimpse—a mere echo—of the resonances of life."[16]

At this writing, the study of the endocrine system gives us a window to the brain, making us spectators at the genesis of psychiatric illness. Let us see what the window shows us of melancholia.

2

Early Days

The brain is the largest of the endocrine organs. In 1987, Philip Gold, head of neuroendocrine research at the National Institute of Mental Health, noted, "It is extraordinary that this concept of the brain as a gland was first advanced in 400 B.C. by Hippocrates, but that so little had been learned about the endocrine functions of the brain over the next 2,350 years."[1] Indeed, for the endocrine functions of the brain to make much impact on psychiatry, it was important to acknowledge that the brain, rather than the mind, is the origin of psychiatric symptoms. The essence of biological psychiatry is dysfunction of the brain.

"Endocrine thinking" does not mark the first eruption of biology into psychiatry, merely the first time that biological psychiatry acquired a scientific basis. But this basis was so shaky that the whole enterprise almost failed.

Before the rise of endocrine thinking, other somatic theories held sway in psychiatry. Reflex theories were prompted in the early nineteenth century by Charles Bell's discovery in 1811 that the posterior roots of the spinal cord connected with the cerebellum.[2] Reflex theory attributed disturbed behavior to pathological reflexes that darted up and down the spine, affecting the brain as well as other organs.[3] Constipation, for example, was thought to create a reflex arc of disease from the colon to the spinal cord to the brain, and in nineteenth-century mental hospitals, patients would often receive a purgative or an enema upon admission. Countless ovaries and uteri were sacrificed in the name of the reflex theory that ovarian "irritation" gave rise to hysteria. Infected teeth were deemed the cause of psychosis, so that mental hospitals often had their own dental laboratories, not to mend caries and rotting teeth, but to extract teeth in hopes of meliorating madness.[4]

Reflex theory sought to make sense of the spinal reflexes, filtered through contemporary prejudices about women and their pelvic organs. But as an explanation of psychopathology, it was inadequate for two reasons: it placed the causative forces in the bodily organs—the uterus, the colon and the teeth—while ignoring the brain. And it was insufficient as an explanation of how parts of the body communicated with one another because it ignored the endocrine system, one of the body's main mechanisms of communication.

In the last third of the nineteenth century, reflex theory was replaced by explanations grounded in neurophysiology. The idea of intrinsic weakness in the brain became dominant. In 1861, Berlin psychiatry professor Wilhelm Griesinger popularized a doctrine of "irritable weakness," or *reizbare Schwäche*, arguing that the more excited or irritable the brain becomes, the less efficiently it performs its functions.[5] The presence of brain commotion and irritable weakness was betrayed by easy exhaustibility or convulsions. In time, neurasthenia became the poster-disease of the irritable weakness model, best exemplified by the image of war neuroses labeled "battle fatigue" and "nervous exhaustion."

Simultaneously, explanations emphasizing the endocrine system were gaining currency. In 1845, John Simon, a surgeon at King's College Hospital in London given to microscopic research in comparative zoology, speculated with great prescience that the thyroid gland lay under cerebral control. The blood chemistry of the day did not give him the means of confirming this suspicion.[6]

Organ transplantations were just beginning in animal research. Endocrinology was founded in 1849 as Arnold Adolph Berthold of the University of Göttingen, Germany, demonstrated that transplanting a rooster's testes to another part of the body prevented atrophy of the comb, otherwise a consequence of castration.[7] This historic work, however, aroused little interest.

Classical accounts of the history of endocrinology begin with the discovery by Thomas Addison, physician at Guy's Hospital in London, of the disease and the anemia that are named after him, occurring in connection with "a diseased condition of the supra-renal capsules," as he explained in 1849.[8] Addison noted the pathology at autopsy and his work did not anticipate the rise of experimental physiology. The establishment of this discipline is instead credited to Claude Bernard, professor of medicine at the Collège de France in Paris. Bernard's ideas on the constancy of the internal environment (*milieu intérieur*) as a precondition for independent life, introduced between 1854 and 1878, were largely ignored during his lifetime, but became a fundamental concept in endocrinology with Walter B. Cannon's introduction of the term *homeostasis* in the 1930s.[9]

Another pioneer of experimental physiology was Charles-Edouard Brown-Séquard. Son of a Philadelphia father and a French mother named Séquard, Brown-Séquard, physician at the National Hospital for the Paralysed and Epileptic in London, in 1856 performed the first experimental adrenalectomies, following which the animals rapidly died. This experiment established the adrenals as essential for life.[10] Neither his nor Addison's work stimulated much attention to the adrenals, however.

"Organ therapy" next caught the attention of the medical profession and the public. In 1889, a flamboyant Brown-Séquard, now professor of experimental physiology in Paris, treated patients with extracts of ground-up testis.[11] At age seventy-one, he injected himself and reported: "I should add that intellectual tasks became easier for me than for some years and that I regained everything that I lost. I must say as well," he added deadpan, "that other forces that were not lost but quite diminished, have considerably improved as well." The following year, 1890, he noted that a female physician in Paris, Dr. Augusta Brown, had cured hysteria with injections of rabbit-ovary extract.[12] But Brown-Séquard's ideas were heavily grounded in reflex theory, and, however forward-looking in principle, aroused laughter in practice. San Francisco endocrinologist Hans Lisser, one-time president of the Endocrine Society, had this to say:

> Pathetically, however, this age-old, old-age striving for the elusive Ponce de Leon fountain of youth, supposedly then achieved by a famous scientist, became a deplorable mirage. [Brown-Séquard's] claims were not confirmed, ridicule and abuse were heaped upon him, and a drought descended upon the field of clinical endocrinology which persisted . . . for almost 30 years. The repercussions from this fiasco caused a cynical eclipse and darkness followed.[13]

The thyroid rather than the testis became the motor of endocrinological progress. Myxedema, a condition involving torpor and a dry, waxy swelling of the skin, is evidence of hypothyroidism. In 1873, Sir William Gull, formerly of Guy's Hospital but now in full-time practice in London, described myxedema in a medical classic: "Miss B., after the cessation of the catamenial period [menopause], became insensibly more and more languid, with general increase of bulk. This change went on from year to year, her face altering from oval to round, much like the full moon at rising." "The mind, which had previously been active and inquisitive, assumed a gentle, placid indifference, corresponding to the muscular languor." What could the faulty organ be, he asked himself? He considered it a kind of cretinism, although the thyroid gland was not enlarged. "But from the folds of skin about the neck, I am not able to state what the exact condition of it was."[14]

In 1890, two investigators in Lisbon, Antonio-Maria Bettencourt-Rodrigues and José-Antonio Serrano, implanted half of a sheep's thyroid gland beneath the breasts of a woman suffering from myxedema.[15] Her symptoms underwent a dramatic improvement, as George Murray, a physician in Newcastle-on-Tyne, speculated a year later, "due to the absorption of the juice of the healthy thyroid gland by the tissues of the patient." Murray thought, "It seems reasonable to suppose that the same amount of improvement might be obtained by simply injecting the juice or an extract of the thyroid gland of a sheep beneath the skin of the patient."[16] This he did in 1891, with spectacular success, becoming, along with the two Portuguese scientists, a founder of endocrinology. It was physiologists William Bayliss and Ernest Starling of University College London who in 1904 adumbrated the concept of hormonal control of internal secretion: a "substance x," secreted in the mucous membrane of the small intestine, was carried to the pancreas.[17] In 1905, Starling coined the term "hormone": "These chemical messengers or 'hormones' . . . as we might call them, have to be carried from the organ where they are produced to the organ which they affect by means of the blood stream."[18]

Endocrine psychiatry did not attract as many adherents as the psychiatry of brain weakness, but it had the advantage of an experimental basis. The findings of endocrine psychiatry were the first convincing accounts of how body processes produce the symptoms of mental illness.

Beginnings of Endocrine Psychiatry

The beginnings of endocrine psychiatry were inauspicious: attributing mental symptoms to the sex organs, especially those of women. In a chapter on "sexual insanity" in 1870, Henry Maudsley, a leading English psychiatrist of his day, said that, "Sexual hallucinations, betraying an ovarian or uterine excitement, might almost be described as the characteristic feature of the insanity of old maids."[19] In 1883, under the pen of Thomas Clouston, professor of psychiatry in Edinburgh, this became "ovarian insanity ('old maid's insanity')": "Out of ten such cases which I can recall, seven had had clergymen as their supposed wooers or seducers. In no case was there the very slightest possible ground for the notion." Delusional erotomania was driven by the ovaries, he thought.[20]

The genital fixation of the early endocrinologists led to one of the unhappiest chapters in the history of medicine: the mass sterilization of young men and women with mental retardation and psychiatric illness in the eugenic era, from around 1890 to the Second World War.[21] Involuntary sterilizations continued apace in Scandinavia and North America into the 1970s.[22] The rationale for these mutilating procedures was genetic rather than endocrine. They were done to avoid infecting the gene pool of coming generations with "bad seed." Nonetheless, it was as a result of an early preoccupation with the testis and ovary that eugenics encountered acceptance.

The founder of *modern* neuroendocrinology, meaning a nonsexual sort that was scientifically verifiable, was the young Parisian physician Maxime Laignel-Lavastine, who wrote a doctoral dissertation on the solar plexus in 1903 and expanded the "sympathetic nervous system" in 1908–1909 to include the adrenal glands, pituitary, thymus, thyroid, parathyroid, testes, and ovaries.[23] Descended from an old family of physicians in Normandy, he was born in 1875 in Évreux, became an "externe" in the Paris hospitals in 1896 and an interne in 1899, and after receiving his M.D. degree in 1903 was trained in internal medicine and psychiatry.[24] His observations were based on both clinical experience and histological findings from numerous autopsies rather than, as in so much scholarship of the day, on reference to the previous literature.

The flurry of work that he published in 1908–1909 represents the first systematic attempt to link the pathological anatomy of the endocrine organs to mental symptoms. Some endocrine conditions with psychiatric sequelae were already familiar. Hyperthyroidism, called "Basedow's disease" (1840), and known in the English world as "Graves' disease," was a cause of nervousness and irritability. Hypothyroidism (myxedema) was associated with depression and psychosis. (The terms "hypothyroidism" and "myxedema" are often used interchangeably.) Addison's disease (1849), or adrenal hypofunction, was similarly familiar. Laignel-Lavastine surveyed the scene of "psycho-glandular relationships,"[25] systematically associating hyper- and hypofunction of the various endocrine organs with mental symptoms. He conceived "endocrine temperaments," and, in addition to the sanguinary and bilious temperaments, he described "the thyroidians, the pituitaries, the adrenals, the ovarians"—all temperaments that determined character.[26]

Laignel-Lavastine argued that "internal secretions" played a big role in "neuropsychiatric" syndromes. He was a vocal advocate of organ therapy, grinding up animal adrenals, thyroids, testes, and ovaries to effect physiological changes in the body and brain.[27] He treated neurasthenia, for example, with thyroid extracts.[28] Of greatest interest was Laignel-Lavastine's attribution of melancholia to the endocrine organs: "It is quite evident that the melancholic syndrome is indeed mental, but simultaneously physical and psychic. It thus seems to me that melancholics are particularly indicated for coming research on endocrine disorders."[29]

The probative value of this work was not great—anecdotally correlating lesions with symptoms that may or may not have been coincidental. The chemistry of endocrinology was in its infancy, and Laignel-Lavastine was not able to demonstrate mechanisms aside from vague invocations of "the sympathetic." But his writing was the groundwork for psychoneuroendocrinology.

In 1939 Laignel-Lavastine was appointed to the chair of psychiatry at the Ste. Anne Mental Hospital in Paris, the summit of French psychiatry. Interestingly, he never embraced the term "endocrine," associating it perhaps with Anglo-Saxon or German scholarship, neither of which languages he customarily cited. He preferred "the sympathetic," or "sympathologie," meaning "the autonomic nervous system."[30] Nor did he evidence much interest in the numerous hormones that had been discovered by the late 1930s. (In fact, he seems to have gone over to homeopathy.[31]) In a sense, he was a figure that psychoneuroendocrinology, a discipline that he had virtually founded, left behind. Yet he did drag the field away from the organs of reproduction toward a scientific assessment of the whole endocrine system.

A Search for Biological Markers of Melancholia

In 1898 William Stoddart, who had trained at the Bethlem Royal Hospital, England's oldest psychiatric hospital, noted a curious physical rigidity in patients with melancholia that disappeared as they got better. "If the nature of this rigidity be examined more closely, it will be found that it is most marked in the muscles of the trunk and neck, that it is less marked but very strikingly present in the muscles of the shoulders and hips," that its presence in the upper limb is diminished, even more so in the lower limb. "I repeat that rigidity of this nature is discoverable in all severe cases of melancholia." Stoddart then proposed a biological marker for the presence of melancholia: "That melancholics are exceedingly tolerant of [pilocarpine]," meaning that they react little to large doses of it. (Pilocarpine, an alkaloid derived from the South American pilocarpus shrub, stimulates the parasympathetic system to produce pupillary contraction, sweating, and salivation, among other symptoms.) Stoddart found it interesting that when he administered pilocarpine to melancholic patients at Bethlem, "the skin was scarcely more than comfortably moist; salivation was not perceptibly increased, nor was there any marked contraction of the pupil." When, by contrast, he administered pilocarpine to himself, he sweated and salivated profusely.

Stoddart carried out a large trial of pilocarpine in patients and controls, measuring perspiration with blotting paper. In twenty-six melancholics, five didn't sweat at all, and for the other twenty-one the average time for onset of sweating was twelve minutes. For the five controls (four patients with other diagnoses plus himself), the average time to sweating was three minutes. One control, a patient with acute mania who had saturated the blotting paper in three minutes, subsequently became melancholic. "This case," said Stoddart, "suggests that the reaction may possibly be useful as a help in diagnosis."[32] He evidently meant that lengthening reaction times would predict the onset of melancholia. Stoddart's pilocarpine reaction test was not picked up in the literature;[33] he himself later lost interest in biological psychiatry and went over to psychoanalysis. But his test appears as the first biological marker for melancholia.

In the years before the First World War, clinical psychoneuroendocrinology galloped ahead in the study of "internal secretions." A role in the causation of psychiatric illness was readily conceded to the thyroid and to underfunctioning adrenals, but this had long been known. It was Harvey Cushing, the American neurosurgeon then at Harvard, who ventured the boldest attempts to connect the endocrine system to the mind. In 1913 he noted that "a primary secretory derangement, in one or the other direction, of each member of the [endocrine gland] series is coupled with its own peculiar and recognizable syndrome." He contrasted the "sympathicotonic individual" (one who secretes readily) with "the vagotonic or more phlegmatic individual ... who responds less readily to the same stimulus." The former might become unnerved under stress and demonstrate glycosuria, exophthalmos, polyuria, and palpitation. Excising the superior cervical ganglion of the sympathetic trunk (which supplies the head and neck) might "diminish an individual's relative sympathicotonicity and lower the threshold of glandular discharge."

The relationship might also run the other way: "It is quite probable that in similar fashion a disorder primarily involving any other member of the ductless gland series leads . . . to an accompanying and character-istic mental change." He pointed to the association of parathyroid tetany with "acute hallucinatory confusion" and to the "characteristic psy-choses" of Addison's disease. He next turned his attention to the pitui-tary gland, with which, as a neurosurgeon, he was quite familiar. The pituitary body, he said, changed considerably during pregnancy, and "it is quite possible that many of the psychoses or insanities associated with this state are coupled with disturbances of the internal secretions." Among his 60 patients with hypopituitarism, "[t]here would seem to be . . . a retardation of mental activity comparable to the lowered meta-bolism of the tissues in general." He also noted the hyperpituitary conditions, which he associated with *dementia praecox* (Kraepelin's term for what was later called schizophrenia).

Cushing warned that Freud's psychoanalysis, which at that point was enveloping psychiatry, viewed things backward, "for the various neuroses and asthenias may arise primarily as the result of some distur-bance of internal secretion which paves the way for the dreams, symbo-lisms, . . . dissected by the psycho-analyst." "It is quite probable that the psychopathology of everyday life [a phrase of Freud's] hinges largely upon the effect of ductless gland discharge upon the nervous system."[34] We are accustomed to think that modern psychoneuroendocrinology took form only in the 1960s. But here, in the writings of this thoughtful neurosurgeon, we see it adumbrated before the First World War.

In those years, German medicine led global science, certainly in psychiatry. Yet the most influential German psychiatric authority, Emil Kraepelin at Munich, was reticent on the psychiatry of the endocrine system. In 1910, in the eighth edition of his influential textbook, Krae-pelin did write of "thyrogenic insanity," then quite a conventional concept. This category became "endocrine insanity" in the posthu-mously published ninth edition in 1927. Kraepelin added a cautionary note: "I am unable to free myself from the thought that the eagerness of researchers to throw light upon an unknown and certainly important area, has in the meantime led to a certain overestimation of the role that the endocrine glands play in mental life."[34] Indeed, it was not the

scientifically meticulous Germans who plunged ahead in linking endocrines to behavior, but investigators in other lands.

The 1920s were the heyday of a physiological psychiatry that is
now largely forgotten. On the therapeutic side, psychiatry buzzed with
endocrine organ-extract therapies. In 1921, Georges Naudascher,
director of a private psychiatric hospital in Évreux near Paris, and his
colleague, Emmanuel Martimor, noted that motor agitation was often
associated with high blood pressure, a result, they said, of a disordered
"sympathique."[36] Two years later, Naudascher found "depressive
states" often in connection with low blood pressure. Therapeutic options
used adrenal organ extracts to reduce blood pressure and adrenalin
(discovered in 1901) to drive it up. [37]

The 1920s again saw a great vogue for treating psychiatric problems
with "spermatogenic" and ovarian extracts. In 1922, Edward Strecker
and Baldwin Keyes at Pennsylvania Hospital in Philadelphia reported
involutional melancholia (melancholia of midlife) much improved after
injections of "ovarian substance." Of fourteen patients, four were
"remarkably improved after an average hospital treatment of seven and
a half months. Four additional patients showed definite improvement,"
and, finally, four remained ill. (One further patient dropped out and
another's response proved difficult to interpret.)[38] In Vienna, psychiatry
professor Julius Wagner-Jauregg developed enthusiasm for sex-organ
treatments of schizophrenia. Some young psychotic patients whose problems, he believed, were associated with delayed onset of puberty were
helped by the administration of "thyroid and ovarian preparations"; as
the secondary sex characteristics developed, the psychosis faltered, and
the patients were discharged. (In some young male patients, whose
schizophrenic symptoms seemed due to "excessive masturbation,"
Wagner-Jauregg offered relief by resecting the vas deferens to sterilize
the lads. Their symptoms improved, and they were able to work again.)[39]

These men were not marginal charlatans but leaders in psychiatry.
Wagner-Jauregg developed the malarial-fever cure for neurosyphilis and
received a Nobel Prize in 1927. In the 1920s there was no grander figure in
French psychiatry than Henri Claude, professor at the Ste. Anne Psychiatric Hospital in Paris. For Claude's psychotic patients, young intern Gilbert
Robin in Claude's service gave the sex hormone androstene in injections
and tablets: "Substantial improvements, outside of any spontaneous remission, have been obtained with this medication."[40]

English physicians in these years set out "to find out if carbohydrate
metabolism is disordered in the different forms of insanity," as Kenneth

Kirkpatrick Drury and C. Farran-Ridge, assistant medical officers at the County Mental Hospital in Stafford, put it in 1925. They said, "Low sugar tolerance is found in melancholia more frequently than in any other psychosis we have examined." The authors concluded "that the general metabolism is far more disordered in insanity than one would be led to believe by casual observation."[41] The conclusions strike us today as rather self-evident, but they were reached in 1925 and then forgotten in the surge toward psychoanalysis.

Interest in the sugar-tolerance test was high in the 1930s, leading László Meduna, who in 1934 originated the concept of convulsive treatments of mental illness, in 1950 to write his treatise *Oneirophrenia*.[42] Meduna applied glucose-tolerance tests to patients whom we would now see as having delirious mania or catatonia. In the same year, he brought out *carbon dioxide therapy*, in which he sought to alter glucose metabolism by inhaled carbon dioxide.[43]

German neuropsychiatrists often attributed an endocrine basis to melancholia. Karl Kleist, originator of the concept of "bipolar disorder" and professor of psychiatry at the University of Frankfurt, speculated in 1921 that the "autochthonous degeneration-psychoses" (by which he meant chronic nonreactive psychoses that did not deteriorate, unlike Kraepelin's dementia praecox) had a large endocrine component. He cited research on breakdown products from the endocrine glands of manic-depressive patients.[44] Kurt Schneider, professor of psychiatry at the University of Cologne, introduced in 1920 the concept of "vital depression,"[45] with an important somatic component, as opposed to reactive depression. In 1922 his student Josef Westermann concluded, "It is conceivable that the basic biological disorder of vital depression, which is certainly to be conceived as endocrine, is similar to the corresponding biological mechanisms that trigger schizophrenia."[46] (This judgment now appears rather prescient, for as we write in the summer of 2009, the National Institute of Mental Health has just issued a press release announcing that "[s]chizophrenia and bipolar disorder share genetic roots." Says Thomas Insel, director of the Institute, "These new results recommend a fresh look at our diagnostic categories."[47])

The Germans also turned to organ therapy, administering extracts of adrenal glands, thyroids, ovaries, or testes orally or as an injection. Melancholia, thought by some German investigators to be the result of heightened sympathetic drive and lessened parasympathetic tone, was treated with the packaged testes-and-thyroid extracts (plus several other ingredients) marketed as "Anermon," to reduce sympathetic tone in male patients.

In females, "Gynormon" (ovarian and thyroid extracts plus other ingredients) was similarly indicated. As far as may be determined from the small number of published cases in open trials, this tactic was quite successful.[48]

The neuropathology school of Karl Schaffer in Budapest was oriented toward Germany, and in 1922, Paul Büchler, a student of Schaffer's, used the phrase "pituitary depression." Several years later he warmed to the theme again, this time with case studies of adrenal disease, concluding, "It is certain that the endocrine apparatus is cerebrally influenced, but also that inversely, endocrine processes can evoke changes in affect." Büchler cited a great raft of European literature that was coming to similar conclusions.[49]

The commercial exploitation of the endocrine therapies was enormous. Glandular extracts, epinephrine and epinephrine-like drugs proliferated in the marketplace. In the late spring of 1913, the pharmaceutical industry offered a veritable harvest of organ-extracts in the pages of the *Vienna Medical Weekly*. Flogged to the medical profession were "Suprarenin of Meister Lucius" by Hoechst am Main, said to be "the synthetically produced active principle of the adrenals";[50] "Antithyreoidin-Moebius" of the Merck Company in Darmstadt, made, according to a standard pharmaceutical guide, "from the serum of thyroidectomized male sheep";[51] and "Pituglandol-Roche," "ten-percent hypophysis [pituitary] extract, presumably successful with amenorrhea, Basedow etc."[52] Rufus McQuillan, sales representative of an unnamed American pharmaceutical company, recalled of the 1920s, "Those were the days of extreme glandular medication." They flogged dried glands, powdered glands, and mixed glands, much like mixed vitamins today: "A mixture would be sure to hit the parts at fault. This glandular medication was accepted by the best doctors in the profession, and they honestly believed they were of great value. We even had Mixed Gland No. 1 and No. 2, male and female respectively."[53] Glandular extracts were big business.

The HPA Axis

The genuine science behind much of this was meager, mostly the systemic and behavioral effects of thyroid and adrenal over- and undersecretion. Boston neurosurgeon Harvey Cushing was not a big fan of the endocrinology of the day; indeed, labeled the quackery-ridden field "endocriminology."[54] But in 1932 Cushing adumbrated the existence of what would later be called a "hypothalamic-pituitary-adrenal" axis with a role in psychiatric illness. At that particular moment, Cushing said nothing about the hypothalamus (which stimulates the lobes of the pituitary gland). But he discovered that the anterior pituitary lobe drove the adrenal gland. In a textbook example of close clinical observation linked to scientific curiosity, Cushing noted that female patients who suddenly became painfully adipose, with amenorrhea and polyuria, and male patients who displayed the same symptoms but whose genitals became hypoplastic, often had small adenomas (tumors) in their anterior pituitary gland. Many would not have been noticed unless sought under the microscope. Such patients would evidence "fits of unnatural irritability alternated with periods of depression." In what later became known as "Cushing's syndrome," Cushing described how a tumor in the anterior pituitary lobe oversecreted substances that drive the endocrine organs of the body, including the adrenal cortex. "Primary adrenal tumors," he wrote, "may cause striking constitutional transformations.... All known primary pituitary disorders inevitably cause marked secondary changes in the adrenal cortex." The makeup of these pituitary and adrenal hormones was as yet unknown. Yet they had the ability to elicit distant changes in the body, such as excessive adiposity. The patients also were depressed and psychotic.[55]

Cushing's discovery established the pituitary-adrenal axis as a mover of psychiatric illness. Awareness of the role of the hypothalamus would come later. Cushing's images were a major scientific accomplishment in a sea of endocrine quackery.

How widespread was endocrine thinking by the 1930s? Quite widespread, although a reaction had already begun to set in.

The young Ralph W. Gerard, then in his mid-thirties, a medical physiologist at the University of Chicago and member of the Chicago neuroscience school, was asked by the Rockefeller Foundation to tour Europe in 1934–1935 to learn what was new and to invite scientists to apply for fellowships. In England, interest in endocrine research was lively. Gerard found Charles P. Symonds, a neurologist at Guy's Hospital and at Queen's Square, to be "a pleasant man in the middle 40s." "Symonds considers that depressions grade all the way into manic-depressive insanity, possibly related to physiological rhythms in the hypo-thalamus."[56] Edward Mapother, director of the Maudsley Hospital in London, "is interested in such problems as: the psychoses of pregnancy, climacteric frigidity, menstrual disturbances in insanity and the like; all of which suggest a definite somatic approach to mental disturbances, possibly via the endocrines."[57] John S. B. Stopford, professor of anatomy at

Manchester, "a small, wizened, energetic man in his middle fifties... thinks many insanities are associated with hypothalamic disturbances."[58]

At the Oslo Psychiatric Hospital in the suburb of Dikemark, Rolf Gjessing, director of the hospital, was in the midst of his important studies on the role of the thyroid in periodic catatonia.[59] Gerard did not see Gjessing himself, but bumped into Dr. Sahtre, the head of psychiatry. "S. finds an excess of pituitary hormone ... in the urine for an indefinite period after gonadectomy and concludes that the gonad hormones have a depressive action on the pituitary and prolan [an undifferentiated reference to luteinizing hormone or follicle-stimulating hormone]." Sahtre was said to have had little success in treating "climacteric insanities" with extracts of various hormones.[60] Elsewhere in Scandinavia, Gerard found an active interest in endocrine psychiatry, albeit of a traditional sort implicating the genitals rather than the hypothalamus and pituitary.

In the world of expensive private clinics, endocrine extract therapy was king. In 1931, Paul Niehans at the Clinique La Prairie in Montreux-Clarens in Switzerland, a private clinic visited heavily by patients with psychoneuroses, began injections of "fresh cells extracted from sheep's fetus" as a revitalization cure. It was apparently the Duke of Windsor who told English novelist Somerset Maugham of the clinic, and in 1938 Maugham, himself a physician and, at 64, his sexual potency waning, checked in for a stay of a few days involving extract injections. "When Niehans examined Maugham," the novelist's biographer tells us, "he complimented him on the youthfulness of his body, the healthy tone of his skin, and the excellent condition of his sexual organs. 'You have lovely soft testicles,'" Niehans told Maugham. Sure enough, after the injections Maugham found himself "with very distinct urges ... usually in the bath."[61] This was an apex, of sorts, for the first phase of endocrine psychiatry.

The Sidelining of Endocrine Psychiatry

Interest in endocrine psychiatry was soon marginalized. In the late 1930s and 1940s, doubts about the role of the endocrines in mental illness gathered among scientists, although less so in community medical practice. In academic circles, the subject became passé.

Ralph Gerard found no endocrine enthusiasts in academic circles in Germany, where doubts began earliest. In 1926, Erich Grafe, professor of internal medicine in Würzburg, said, "There was a time—and it's scarcely over and some believe we're still in the midst of it—in which more or less all metabolic disorders were reducible to endocrine disorders. As far as I can see, this endocrine era in medicine, that we in Germany and Austria have experienced in especially strong measure, is dying out. And rightly so." Grafe viewed the central nervous system as taking over from the endocrines with Otto Loewi's discovery of a "vagus-hormone." [62] (In 1921, Loewi, in Graz, discovered acetylcholine, the first of the neurotransmitters.)

German academic psychiatrists showed themselves just as disillusioned as the internists—or almost. Paul Schmidt, a former student of Karl Kleist and now at the university psychiatric clinic in Osnabrück, noted in 1928 that endocrine psychiatry had more or less run into the sand. But Ciba's corpus-luteum preparation "Agomensin," he said, did seem to have an elective effect on schizophrenia when the disease was associated with the ovaries.[63] (The idea here was that supposed ovarian influences on the brain might cause insanity. In 1932 another Kleist student, Herbert Sack, also saw some benefit in using ovarian preparations in women with constitutional depressions, unlike melancholia.[64] Although Sack was quite enthusiastic about this approach, German psychiatrists were not receptive.)

When Munich psychiatry professor Oswald Bumke brought out his multivolume compendium on mental illness at the end of the 1920s—which at once became the authoritative account worldwide—Otto Wuth at the University of Munich, who wrote the section on body weight and metabolic and endocrine disorders, gave the endocrine side of things the back of his hand.

> After the role of the thyroid gland became apparent in the clinical pictures of myxedema and cretinism, and affections of psychic activity seemed to be reducible to the dysfunction of a single endocrine organ, it was only natural that people would draw parallel conclusions about the etiology of almost all psychotic and neurotic reactions. It is clear that this has led to widely overshooting the target. The results have in no way conformed to the expectations.[65]

The final death knell of old-style endocrine psychiatry—associating microscopic lesions with behavioral disorders without an intervening biochemical link—was sounded in 1954 by Manfred Bleuler, professor of psychiatry at the University of Zurich, whose father, Eugen Bleuler, a generation previously had occupied the same chair. On the causation side, Bleuler called the relationship between mental life and the endocrine system "a puzzle"—little was understood. On the treatment side, he said, "In view of earlier failures and transgressions and of the inadequacy of our knowledge, it's my conviction that endocrine psychiatry today has the duty to warn about 'too much' rather than beating the drums for 'still more'—even though this runs the risk of disappointing many." He deplored the orgy of endocrine surgical interventions that had been done in the name of psychiatry: "massive castrations in schizophrenia, epilepsy, hysteria, psychopathy; thyroidectomies for schizophrenia, manic-depressive illness . . . . Extirpation of the adrenals for epilepsy, schizophrenia and affective psychoses; the Steinach operations [a vasectomy to restore youth], and further organ implantations of the most varied kind." As for organ extract therapy, he said, "The chain of the most diverse hormone preparations for the most diverse psychiatric disorders is endless. It would not be exaggerated to maintain that almost every organ extract of the inner glands and almost every isolated hormone has been tried in the course of the last seventy years for almost every mental disorder (which is praiseworthy) and also recommended (which is often much less praiseworthy)."[66]

In addition to sheer failure in efficacy, the fateful association with the organs of reproduction also dragged down early endocrine psychiatry, especially the reproductive organs of women, an inheritance of male prejudices against women stretching back to time out of mind. The link between ovaries and mental illness became increasingly questionable in scientific terms and socially *démodé* as well. "Endocrinology suffered obstetric deformity at its very birth," said one wag after the formation of the United States "Association for the Study of Internal Secretions" in 1917.[67] Estrogen does not seem to work as an antidepressant in menopausal women, concluded a team from the New York Hospital in 1940, a team that included George Papanicolaou (originator of the "Pap" smear for cervical cancer).[68]

Endocrine psychiatry became something of a joke. When James Collip, chair of biochemistry at McGill University in Montreal, whose team had isolated ACTH in 1933, gave Heinz Lehmann, chief psychiatrist at the Douglas Hospital in Montreal, a supply of pituitary extract to try in schizophrenia, Lehmann believed the patient had improved mainly because the extract had a high alcohol content.[69]

Under these circumstances, one would have said that endocrine psychiatry, like other medical holdovers from the nineteenth century such as bleeding for fever, was dead.

3

Cortisol

The drama of endocrine psychiatry is the drama of cortisol: its discovery, synthesis, and role in psychiatric illness.

The Discovery of the Adrenal Cortex Steroids

Tadeus Reichstein was born in Poland in 1897. His family was poor and moved often. Living with an aunt in Lublin in 1905, he was horrified at the violence of a pogrom he witnessed and was sent to a brutal German boarding school for two years. Finally, in the spring of 1907, his father succeeded in buying a house on the outskirts of Zurich, reuniting the family. Reichstein studied at a technical high school and then entered the State Technical College (the German initials of which are ETH), earning a doctorate in 1922 under Hermann Staudinger and learning the ins and outs of organic chemistry under Staudinger's assistant, Leopold Ruzicka.

From 1922 to 1931, under Staudinger's guidance, Reichstein, assisted by Joseph von Euw, worked at a small private laboratory isolating volatile components in roasted coffee. In 1931 he returned to ETH as a university lecturer and Ruzicka's assistant at the Organic Chemical Institute. Reichstein synthesized vitamin C two years later in 1933, considered by his biographer, Miriam Rothschild, to be "the foundation stone for the modern bridge spanning organic chemistry and medicine."[1] It was the capstone of his career.

When Reichstein won an associate professorship in 1934, he and his assistant (and lifelong friend), von Euw, turned to the composition of the hormones in the adrenal cortex, or outer layer of the adrenal gland. Experimentally removing the adrenal cortex was fatal to laboratory cats and dogs. The adrenal medulla (center) produced adrenalin. But what life-sustaining substance did the cortex produce?

A number of teams in chemistry departments across the Atlantic community sought to extract the active principle from the adrenal cortex in the late 1920s and early 1930s. Some researchers spoke of the "adrenal cortex hormone,"[2] but Reichstein ultimately determined that there were twenty-eight different extracts. Six had an active "corticoid" effect in the body. One was cortisone, which a competing group at the Mayo Clinic in Rochester, Minnesota, led by Edward Kendall, had isolated in 1935 and which Reichstein also discovered in 1936. Cortisone became hugely important in medical therapeutics.

But another member of this series of steroid hormones on which both Reichstein and Kendall were working differed very slightly from cortisone: at position "eleven" on the molecule of this other steroid (called Substance "M" by Reichstein and Compound "F" by Kendall), there was an "OH," or hydroxy, molecule rather than a carbon-oxygen (carbonyl) molecule. Substance M, too, was one of the six, but nobody paid particular attention to it in 1937 when Reichstein discovered it.[3] This was cortisol.

Cortisol is the more important adrenal cortex hormone for our purposes and predominates among the circulating adrenocorticoids. It plays a capital role in psychiatry, because the adrenal gland hypersecretes cortisol in melancholia. It is a biological marker of melancholic depression. Not all melancholias show elevated cortisol levels, but enough do to raise the question: What is distinctive about this biologically homogeneous group of melancholic depressives?

Aggressive Endocrinology

In the late 1930s, these newly isolated corticosteroids were available only in tiny amounts and insufficient for therapeutic use. But the very fact that the hormones of the adrenal cortex had been isolated revived curiosity about endocrinology in psychiatry. It offered fresh promise for understanding psychiatric illness. Active preparations of adrenal cortex extract (all 28 hormones mixed together) were marketed in the 1930s. In 1937, an adrenal cortical extract highly purified by Wilbur Swingle and Joseph Pfiffner was patented as "Eschatin" by Parke Davis & Company in Detroit.[4] Adrenal cortex extracts entered psychiatric treatment.

In 1938, psychiatrist Conrad Loehner in Salem, Oregon, treated various mental illnesses with adrenal cortex extract. After injecting 10 cc intramuscular into patients, he wrote in 1940: "The mood changes to euphoria and elation; a feeling of warmth suffuses the body, especially the extremities which are often cyanotic and cold. Shortly afterwards the patient has a marked desire to sleep, and upon wakening he is refreshed and alert." One hypomanic patient had not done well with bromides, so Loehner injected her with the extract. A few days later, "her mental symptoms disappeared." In schizophrenia, Loehner's results were impressive. A twenty-one-year-old woman with dementia praecox of the "hebephrenic" variety "complained of loss of interest, inability to concentrate and loss of memory. She was silly, indifferent and emotionally inadequate." Over two months, Loehner gave her 60 cc of extract: "Her mental symptoms disappeared and she has remained well for over a year." He reported similar results in an endocrinology journal, eschewing a psychiatry journal, as these were the years when psychiatry was overwhelmed by psychoanalysis.[5]

Desoxycorticosterone, or Doca, one of the six active fractions of adrenal cortex hormone, was the earliest fraction available in pure form; Reichstein synthesized it in 1937 from a cholesterol derivative, and Ciba brought it out in 1939 as an oily injection for patients with Addison's disease.[6] Following Loehner's good results with psychosis, in 1941 Harry Haynes and Chester Carlisle at the Veterans Administration Hospital in Palo Alto, California, injected desoxycorticosterone acetate into some of their chronic catatonic "schizophrenic" patients, men in the hospital since World War I. (With some "schizophrenia" reports, the patients may well have had catatonia or psychotic depression, conditions that might respond more favorably to steroid treatment.[7]) The authors theorized that the pressor effect of the adrenocorticoids raising the blood pressure might act favorably upon the illness: "The blood pressure rose approximately 10 mm of mercury in both the systolic and diastolic pressure, and there was a transitory reversal of the mood to mild euphoria and elation, in one case. In all cases there was a feeling of warmth, drowsiness, and general relaxation."[8] Clinical improvement was maintained, and the blood pressure remained elevated.

These early successes revived interest in endocrine psychiatry, similar to the pre-World War I thinking of Laignel-Lavastine, who argued that when endocrine disorders and mental problems occur together, the one has clearly caused the other. But in the early 1940s, powerful new extracts of pituitary, adrenal, testis, corpus luteum, and ovary became available, encouraging more refined testing than had been possible before.

At the center of this work were the mental hospitals of Bristol, England, particularly the Burden Neurological Institute, where Max Reiss, an émigré medical biochemist from Prague, directed the Endocrinological Department. Reiss began his endocrine research at the Burden in 1940, coauthoring with Yolande Golla, also at the Institute, an article on the endocrines and cerebral blood supply in the rat (sex hormones seem to increase the blood content.)[9]

Reiss's associate in much of this work, Robert Hemphill, was director of clinical services in the Bristol Mental Hospital. Hemphill had been drawn to endocrinology in 1940, working with Vienna émigré psychiatrist Erwin Stengel on what was known at the time as "Morgagni's syndrome"—later called *hyperostosis frontalis interna*, "Morel's syndrome," or "Morgagni-Stewart-Morel syndrome"—a thickening of the frontal bones of the skull occurring mainly in women and characterized by endocrine changes of obesity, hirsutism, and psychiatric disturbances.[10] Hemphill and Stengel thought the syndrome might be of endocrine origin, the result of a pituitary adenoma. (It is striking how much of this British research was spark-plugged by fleeing Jewish refugees; in other centers, such figures as Willy Mayer-Gross and Eric Guttmann provided scholarly leadership for an entire generation of British psychiatrists.)

In 1942, Hemphill, building upon Gjessing's work on "periodic catatonia," studied the relationship between thyroid overactivity and mental illness. He found none, with the exception of toxic goiter (hyperthyroid) related to a form of catatonia found in "schizophrenia." Gjessing assumed that his periodic-catatonia patients were hypothyroid, because administration of thyroxin resolved the nitrogen retention thought to be the cause of catatonia. Hemphill, in research that was never really picked up—perhaps because of the war—found the exact opposite: "hyperthyrotic catatonia."[11]

Hemphill and Reiss began their collaboration in the war years and continued for the next two decades.

Some of their research was of the traditional variety, such as incriminating menopause as a cause of psychiatric disorder and treating involutional melancholia, or midlife depression, by prescribing steroids to menopausal women. In 1944, Hemphill wrote that involutional melancholia was presumably caused by "hypopituitarism with inadequate output of corticotrophic hormone." The women at midlife had "asthenia...cutaneous pigmentation, brittle hair, low blood pressure...combined with anorexia, delusions of alimentary disorder, and severe melancholic depression.... Treatment with a purified biologically active corticotrophic hormone brought about improvement in appetite and general physical condition with loss of the specific delusions of visceral illness."[12]

The Bristol work did not just entail medicating menopause. Reiss and Hemphill also treated the "male climacteric" with testosterone. Anorexia nervosa was attributed to "hypopituitarism" (Simmonds' disease), and, "if 17-keto-steroid output is low," corticotrophic hormone was offered. (17-Keto-steroids are metabolites mainly of adrenal steroids; they are found in the urine). Hemphill wrote in 1944, "In no psychosis...can endocrine abnormalities be demonstrated as readily and with such a diversity of form as in schizophrenia." Furthermore, "[a]nxiety and a sense of impending disaster" might announce hypoparathyroidism, while suprarenal extract might clear up "confusional insanity." In homosexuality, "[t]here is...striking evidence that an endocrine abnormality exists in some forms of homosexuality.... There is no known endocrine treatment."[13] These propositions might be hotly contested today, but they illustrate the extent to which a new psychoneuroendocrinology, centered upon treatment, not microscopy, was spreading in the 1940s.

The new psychiatric endocrinology gave rise to Oxford psychiatrist Tayleur Stockings' diagnosis of "thalamic dysfunction" for the entire spectrum of depression, anxiety, and obsessive-compulsive disorder—what might be called today "nonmelancholic mood disorder."[14] Stockings wrote in 1947, "The essential feature common to all of these disorders is a condition of the nervous system in which the perception-threshold for unpleasant affects and sensory impressions is markedly lowered, while that for pleasant affect and sensation is correspondingly raised—the anhedonic or dysphoric syndrome." The cause? "Although it is generally taught at the present day that these conditions are entirely psychogenic in origin, there would appear to be strong evidence that the basis of the condition is primarily a disturbance of the thalamic-hypothalamic mechanisms, possibly a metabolic disorder." Thus, according to Stockings, most outpatient psychiatry was reducible to dysfunction in the endocrine system.[15] Few diagnosticians adopted the concept of a "thalamic dysfunction syndrome." Yet it anticipated the findings of later research. Stockings' proposal of thalamic dysfunction foreshadows today's focus on cortico-striato-thalamo-cortical circuits in mood disorder, and his observation of altered thresholds for pleasant and unpleasant affects and sensations foreshadows what is now called the Carroll-Klein model of mood disorder.[16] The original outline of this model was first articulated by Donald F. Klein and John M. Davis in their 1969 textbook on drug treatment in psychiatry.[17]

As these events transpired—mainly in the United Kingdom, for war-torn Europe was silent and the United States was engulfed in psycho-analysis—an émigré physician in Montreal was preparing a quite dif-ferent justification for endocrine interventions in psychiatry. Hans Selye popularized the concept of "stress." Born in Vienna in 1907, Selye graduated in medicine from the German University of Prague in 1929 and, after earning a doctorate in experimental pathology, received a Rockefeller scholarship to come to Johns Hopkins University. In 1932 he settled in Montreal as a lecturer in biochemistry at McGill University. In experiments to which serendipity drove him, he noted adrenal enlar-gement in rats that had been subject to various stressors such as cold.[18] In 1936, at age twenty-nine, Selye published in *Nature* the first of an ava-lanche of articles on the impact of "stress" on the body.[19] (*Stress* was a term Harvard physiologist Walter Cannon had used medically as early as 1914, if not before, and it was Cannon who put on the medical radar the consequences of stressful actions upon the glands and the autonomic nervous system, which he captured with the phrase "fight or flight."[20])

Stress produced a characteristic enlargement of the adrenals and a discharge of cortisol following stimulation of the pituitary gland. "This suggested," Selye wrote in 1950, "that perhaps in man also all the systemic diseases, indeed all the stresses and strains of normal life, are met by a similar defensive corticoid production."[21] Some authorities consider Selye to have launched the rebirth of endocrinology.[22] Yet Selye had little time for Tadeus Reichstein and Harvey Cushing, who are barely glimpsed in his enormous bibliography that heavily features his own writing. His fame represents a triumph of self-promotion more than of science. One of his students, Roger Guillemin—who later shared a Nobel Prize for discovering the structure of TRH—wrote of his own years in Montreal, "I had come to recognize that Selye's style was absolutely unique and probably not to be emulated. It would always be dealing with a purely descriptive phenomeno-logy, with more than a touch of the dramatic and a quasi-paranoid need to be read and/or presented as generating unified theories of medicine."[23]

Also, some psychiatrists were unhappy that Selye reduced the panoply of psychiatric illnesses to "stress." Seymour Levine, a Stanford University psychiatrist, said in 1984, "Hans Selye left us with a horrible legacy: the legacy that equated stress and disease—and with a set of interwoven nuances with little or no data."[24] Selye's general adaptation syndrome bypassed most of psychoneuroendocrinology and jumped straight to philosophizing about the human condition. Still, Selye's work focused attention on the endocrine system as the mediator between external events and internal lesions.

Cortisol and Depression

Psychiatry already had several biological tests of disease. In 1905, August Wassermann, a staff physician at Robert Koch's Institute for Infectious Diseases at the Charité Hospital in Berlin, described a diagnostic test for neurosyphilis based on complement fixation in the cerebrospinal fluid. After Hans Berger, professor of psychiatry in Jena, described EEG in 1929, it was not long before it became, in 1935, a biological test for epilepsy (in those days in the province of neuropsychiatry).[25] So even before the advent of interest in the adrenal cortex, psychiatry did possess useful biological markers. But in the large arena of mood disorders there were few.

In the background are the great strides that biochemistry made after the Second World War, replacing the microscope with the chemistry laboratory to examine changes in brain and body. The method for detecting adrenal cortex hormones in the urine (ketosteroids) that Zimmermann described in 1935 was capable of separating various steroids with $CO-CH_2$ (ketone) groups.[26] Nancy Callow and co-workers at Middlesex Hospital in London improved the method somewhat in 1939,[27] and the Bristol group led by Max Reiss improved it further.

These technical advances led to the first biochemically based efforts to associate corticosteroids with psychiatric illness. In 1949, Reiss and Hemphill conducted a controlled experiment, giving one group of chronic schizophrenics in the Bristol Mental Hospital dehydroepiandrosterone, a steroid hormone midway on the pathway between cholesterol (where the pathway begins) and testosterone. (An alternative pathway leads from cholesterol to cortisol.) To another group of chronic schizophrenics they administered a pituitary extract containing a heavy mixture of gonadotropic hormone (the pituitary hormones are peptides and glycoproteins, which are smaller than steroids with their distinctive ring system). The investigators were quite surprised when they found that urinary output of 17-ketosteroid rose in the dehydroepiandrosterone group. By contrast, the control group receiving the pituitary extract saw a decline in their urinary 17-ketosteroid excretion. Reiss and Hemphill were puzzled: There was something about injecting an exogenous steroid that increased the level of adrenal corticoid secretion.[28] Was this in everybody or only in those who were ill?

Meanwhile, in the United Sates, a small corps of psychiatrists had escaped the pull of psychoanalysis and continued to undertake biological studies. At the newly created Institute for Psychobiological Studies at Creedmoor State Hospital in New York, Johan H. W. van Ophuijsen had just joined the Sackler brothers—Arthur, Mortimer, and Raymond, all psychiatrists—in what was probably the first American center devoted to endocrine psychiatry. Van Ophuijsen wrote in 1951 that the pendulum had swung too far toward psychoanalysis and that it was time to swing back "in the direction of physical phenomena and probably of biochemical disturbances in particular." The team at the Creedmoor Institute had endocrinology in mind.[29] They picked up on the English and European tradition, dating from the early 1940s, of treating psychiatric patients with hormones, especially testosterone.[30]

Indeed, testosterone treatments of psychosis, especially schizophrenia, lingered on into the 1950s in Czechoslovakia. In Prague, internist Joseph Marek was impressed by the Sacklers' contributions on endocrine treatment of psychoses. Marek, who declared that "psychopharmacology is the endocrinology of the brain," treated psychotic young women with estrogen in order to reduce cortisol levels.[31]

Other endocrine hormones shone in the spotlight as well. Even though an impure form of ACTH—secreted by the pituitary to activate the adrenals—had been isolated by Collip in 1933,[32] only in 1943 did Choh Hao Li and co-workers at the Institute of Experimental Biology of the University of California at Berkeley isolate a pure form of ACTH from sheep pituitary glands.[33] Armour put a commercial form on the market around 1946, and in the early 1950s, different groups began treating illnesses such as Guillain-Barré syndrome with it.[34] In 1951, Howard P. Rome and Francis J. Braceland in the Department of Neurology and Psychiatry of the Mayo Clinic described the psychological response to ACTH, cortisone, hydrocortisone, and other steroids: "Cortisone and ACTH as potent pharmacological agents are prone . . . to jeopardize a precarious stability by depriving the patient of the keystone of his psychological defense. This, coupled with their ability to modify ego defenses, is often sufficient to precipitate an acute psychological decompensation."[35] Two years later, Arthur Mirsky, who had just arrived in Pittsburgh as chair of the Clinical Science department—and who had been psychoanalyzed—noted the effect of ACTH upon the behavior of monkeys. (He was aided in this by a young psychiatrist, Marvin Stein, who would end up as longstanding chair of psychiatry at Mt. Sinai Hospital in New York.)[36]

Yet little of psychiatric interest was discovered with ACTH, except that it could elicit delirious states.[37] One negative finding, however, was worth filing away, not because of the finding but because of the question behind it. Could there be differential responsiveness by diagnosis to injected ACTH? Looking at 17-ketosteroid excretion in urine, Reiss and Hemphill in 1951 found no difference in response to ACTH injections among chronic schizophrenia, acute schizophrenia, depression, or anxiety states. "There was no appreciable difference in the distribution of extreme types of response to ACTH in the different disease groups," the authors said.[38] But the question was planted: might other agents demonstrate differential responsiveness by disease?

During the Second World War, there was great interest in the corticosteroids for increasing the endurance of troops. In a government crash program, several chemists of the Merck Company, including Lewis Sarett, came to Rochester, Minnesota, to work in Kendall's Mayo laboratory.[39] As well, in the world of steroid treatment there was curiosity about cortisone (Kendall's Compound E). In 1946, Sarett developed a synthesis that yielded large amounts;[40] it was first put into a patient with arthritis at Mayo in 1948, and in 1950 Merck marketed cortisone as Cortone Acetate. (In 1949, Kendall and Mayo clinician Philip Hench, both of whom shared a Nobel Prize with Reichstein in 1950, coined the term "cortisone."[41])

Because cortisone and cortisol are almost chemical twins, the cortisone boom drew interest toward "cortisol" as well, a term that Charles W. Shoppee at the University of Wales, Swansea—a British-born biochemist who worked as Rockefeller Research Fellow at Basel University with Reichstein during World War II—coined in 1953 for what Reichstein had called 17-hydrocorticosterone.[42] Cortisol became available for clinical use in 1950 when Norman L. Wendler and Max Tishler at Merck developed its synthesis.[43] On the basis of a

color-reaction test that Porter and Silber had developed in 1950,[44] Don
Nelson and Leo Samuels at the University of Utah College of Medicine
worked out a technique in 1952 involving chromatography and color-
reaction for determining the level of adrenal steroids in the blood.[45]
This small technical innovation opened up the study of cortisol in
psychiatry.

In 1954, psychiatrist Eugene Bliss at Utah, together with endocrinologist colleagues, studied the blood concentration of cortisol in psychiatric illness and controls. They found that stress and emotional upset
greatly increased blood levels of cortisol in psychiatric patients. The 267
normal subjects had a cortisol level of 13 micrograms per 100 cc plasma;
the 19 disturbed psychiatric patients had a level of 22 micrograms per 100
cc, a highly significant difference. By contrast, the 8 calm psychiatric
patients, mostly chronic schizophrenics who, the authors felt, had little
to be anxious or tense about, had the same cortisol blood levels as the
normal subjects. The authors did not home in on depression, but this is
the first solid indication that cortisol was elevated in specific forms of
psychiatric illness rather than just being an effect of "stress."[46] The results
also indicated that ambient stress or distress is capable of increasing
plasma cortisol concentrations. Exactly the same response would be
seen in the 1990s in the public-speaking task known as the Trier Social
Stress Test.[47]

A quickening of interest in cortisol, marketed by Merck in 1952
as hydrocortisone, took place against a background of rising therapeutic curiosity about steroid treatments. The quickening of interest
would be brief. The First World Congress of Psychiatry in Paris in
1950 prominently featured an endocrine session. Diogo Furtado of
Lisbon gave an overview of endocrine treatments that concentrated
on ACTH and desoxycorticosterone (the precursor of corticosterone)
to elevate blood pressure. Cortisone and ACTH, he said, also had an
independent effect on psychosis.[48] Analogizing from the stimulating
effect of ECT upon the adrenal cortex, Max Reiss and Robert
Hemphill from Bristol took a closer look at the pituitary in psychiatric illness. They argued for the administration of ACTH to stimulate the adrenal cortex when response tests showed that depressed
and schizophrenic patients were underproducing their own ACTH
and corticosteroids.[49]

The steroids enjoyed their brief moment in psychiatric treatment.
At the Second International Congress of Psychiatry in Zurich in 1957, a
team of university psychiatrists in Poitiers, France, said that they gave

serotonin to treat "inertia, apathy, and athymia," augmenting it with androstanolone "in heavy doses," an anabolic steroid synthesized in 1935 from a precursor of testosterone. "This is a psychotonic steroid," they said, "that stimulates the appetite and the general state of health and may render service in case of anorexia."[50]

Nor were psychiatric endocrine interventions confined to medication. Under the direction of Hudson Hoagland at the Worcester Foundation for Experimental Biology at Shrewsbury, Massachusetts, and in collaboration with surgeon Charles Huggins at the University of Chicago (who won a Nobel Prize in 1966 for his work on hormones and prostate cancer), six patients with schizophrenia either at the Billings Hospital in Chicago or the Worcester State Hospital, were experimentally adrenalectomized, then maintained on cortisone or hydrocortisone, to study the relationship between adrenals and psychosis. "Unfortunately we were unable to find any consistent changes in the personalities following adrenalectomy," Hoagland reported in 1956. "If one adrenalectomizes and maintains these people on cortisone it might be expected that the abnormal steroid substances, if present, would thus be eliminated and this might have therapeutic value. But adrenalectomy did not produce significant improvement in the patients" (although it might have raised the eyebrows of subsequent generations of bioethicists).[51]

In the late 1950s the corticosteroid markets in internal medicine, family practice, and other fields were aroused. Many firms rushed in with new products, threatening the sales primacy of Merck's cortisone and hydrocortisone and Schering's prednisone (Meticorten) and prednisolone (Meticortelone). By 1958, these companies, which had dominated the nascent steroid market since the launch of cortisone in 1950, were giving ground to Squibb and Lederle's triamcinolone (Kenacourt, Aristocort).[52]

But in psychiatry, the steroids were seeping out of clinical practice in these years with the advent of new, effective forms of pharmacotherapy appeared, such as chlorpromazine, an antipsychotic, which was launched in 1954, and imipramine, an antidepressant, in 1959. It looked as though a page was being turned on the therapeutic side of endocrine psychiatry, in vogue for the prior twenty years.

There was one other relevant event in 1958. In October of that year, the U.S. FDA gave marketing approval to Decadron, Merck's new artificial steroid, introduced to reinforce the firm's flagging share of the market. The generic term for Decadron was dexamethasone.

A Test for Depression

In 1955, Francis Board, who had just finished a residency in psychiatry at the Institute for Psychosomatic and Psychiatric Research and Training of Michael Reese Hospital in Chicago, and David Hamburg, associate director of the Institute, began taking blood samples of patients admitted to the unit. For thirty patients whom they interviewed the day after admission, they took one sample at 9:00 A.M., another at noon, and a third around two weeks after admission. The patient group was "considerably weighted on the side of mild and moderate degrees of emotional disturbances," where the patients were able to cooperate. There were twenty-four normal individuals as controls. Although the psychosomatic unit at Michael Reese Hospital was interested in psychoanalysis, neither Board nor Hamburg had trained in analysis (though Board would do so later). Hamburg, in fact, had done a two-year stint in the Army from 1950 to 1952 at Fort Sam Houston in Texas and would have observed the somatic treatments of electroshock and insulin coma.

Using the Nelson-Samuels blood test, they found that the average plasma level of cortisol for patients was 19.8 micrograms per 100 cc of plasma and 12.3 for normal controls. The difference was highly significant. These findings did not go beyond that of the Bliss study at the University of Utah two years previously. What did break new ground was their analysis of corticosteroids by diagnosis.

Table 3.1 Blood Adrenocortical Hormone Levels of Newly Admitted Psychiatric Patients, By Diagnostic Classification

Psychotic depressives	22.2 (significantly higher than in normals in p value)
All psychotics	20.8 (significantly higher than in normals)
Schizophrenics	18.1 ($n = 5$, too few to analyze)
All neurotics	17.1 (significantly higher than in normals)
Neurotic depressives	16.4 (significantly higher than in normals)

Psychotic depression was at one end of the scale, neurotic depression at the other. This suggested strongly that psychotic depression, a form of melancholia, was a biologically different entity than neurotic depression, the "walking wounded" of the psychoanalytic world.

The investigators also found that, in the course of hospitalization, as the patients improved, the average cortisol level for the fourteen patients who remained in the unit longer than two weeks dropped from 17.2 at admission to 11.5 at discharge, a significant decline.[53] Yet, riveting though these findings appear in retrospect, they aroused a deep yawn in the mid-1950s. They were little commented on, and no one attempted a replication.[54]

The scene shifted to the Maudsley Hospital in London, where, seven years later, in 1962, James Gibbons, a senior lecturer in the Department of Psychiatry, and the young American Paul McHugh, a visiting fellow on a National Institutes of Health (NIH) fellowship, collaborated on a biochemical study of depression. What happened to cortisol levels in seventeen depressed patients who were followed longer than two weeks? They determined cortisol levels by the method originated by Ralph Peterson at the NIH in 1957 (modified by others two years later).[55] And they undertook a careful evaluation of the degree of depression. They found a smooth correlation between the severity of depression and the level of plasma cortisol: the worst-depressed had a cortisol level of 26.3 micrograms per 100 ml and the least depressed 9.5, with regularly descending gradations in between. The number of subjects was admittedly small, but these data made depression look like a disease of cortisol!

Gibbons and McHugh also confirmed the Michael Reese observation that cortisol levels fell as patients improved. Of the forty-six clinical ratings in patients who improved, cortisol levels dropped in 63 percent. Of the fifty-four ratings in patients who failed to get better, cortisol dropped in only 33 percent (and rose in 30 percent).[56] Of this historic work in psychiatric endocrinology, McHugh later said in an interview[57]:

> During my doctoral degree in science, I arrived at the Maudsley to work with James [Gibbons], and he said, "There have been some suggestions already about the adrenal cortex and depression, and we're going to start measuring cortisol in the blood."
>
> I said, "Well, how do we do that?" and he said, "Here's how it's measured, here's the article on the contemporary method."
>
> So I said, "Okay, we'll do it."
>
> "*You'll* do it!" (*laughter*)
>
> He says, "Read this." So I started reading it, and I set up the cortisol method, and I learned an awful lot, including how you have to wash the glassware, and in the process spoiled several ties by spilling acid on the ties to get the glassware absolutely pristine acid-cleaned—and then did everything. I went and interviewed the cases. I went and drew the blood. I took the blood back to the laboratory, I measured the levels. I collected the data, and saw the cases on the metabolic unit. Some of them were on the metabolic unit of the Maudsley, some of them were on the main wards of the Maudsley. But under James's direction, I fundamentally did everything....

We found an elevation of the plasma cortisol that correlated very directly with the severity of the depression in the patients that we were seeing. As well, we saw—because we had a wonderful bipolar patient, or a manic patient—that every time she got sick, she got manic, her plasma cortisols fell, and every time she got depression, her plasma cortisols went up.

McHugh said that the research experience with Gibbons marked his passage from neurology, which he had studied at the Peter Bent Brigham Hospital in Boston, to psychiatry. He continued (about how he had reached the Maudsley),

At the Brigham, George Thorn [physician-in-chief] told me, "If you go in the direction that everybody is going in psychiatry here in Boston [psychoanalysis], you are going to be in a dead end. You're not going to play with the big boys. I don't know whether you want to do this, but if you want to, you have to approach psychiatry first through training in neurology." This was before the word "neuroscience" crossed anybody's mind. So I ended up with Ray Adams at the Mass General. [Adams was professor of neurology and author of the standard textbook.]

Ray Adams said, "Okay, we'll teach you neurology, but then you're going to have to do psychiatry with a kind of endocrine bent, because you've come out of the Brigham," and he said, "The place for you to go is the Maudsley."

He called Aubrey Lewis [professor of psychiatry at the Maudsley] and said, "I've got this bright kid, and he's now finishing his training here." Aubrey said, "Have him come over." I got an NIH fellowship to go there. And because I was kind of "von Adams," they attached me to the endocrine-metabolic unit to get my training at the Maudsley in psychiatry.

Then McHugh made a mistake, as he put it, with portentous consequences for the rest of his career (he was for many years the chair of psychiatry at the Johns Hopkins University School of Medicine):

The only mistake I made in my life, and it was a big mistake, was that I decided I had to go off and do basic science. I left the Maudsley, and went to the Walter Reed after this paper [with Gibbons] was finished, because I wanted to learn something about the hypothalamus and the limbic system. I should have stayed. If I had stayed at the Maudsley, we would have gone on. The next step was to do the dexamethasone suppression test and things of that sort, and to see in which ways various people in various states of mind could be shown. That's how it all came about, and it was wonderful. It was the best experience in science that I had had in my life up to that time.

Was Eugene Bliss's above-mentioned work much help?

Not much. We knew that there was something there. Bliss's paper said that there might be something there, and he emphasized the issue of stress. But he didn't have the graded form [of evaluating depression], and he didn't go after it in relationship even to a bipolar phenomenon. We went after it. I've got to tell you, Max [Fink], when I started off, I had the sense that we were going to be kind of like Bliss, never quite certain as to what we had identified, and as these data started coming in—it was amazing to me. Holy Catfish! . . . . The files as to how depressed I thought they were, in a kind of crude depressive rating, were in one set, and the [lab] values were all coming out somewhere else. It was only when we started putting them together, we said, "Holy smoke! Look, they add up." It was an eye-opening experience about empirical research.

This cortisol research touched off a great deal of excitement in psychiatry and in endocrinology. Psychiatry, hitherto dependent on utterances from "the couch," now had the chance of establishing a physiological base even more solid than that which psychopharmacology was laying down. There were no biological tests in psychopharmacology for how ill a patient was: Cortisol, which is to say 17-hydroxycorticosteroid, was unique as a marker. In 1964, Howard Kurland, in the Neuropsychiatric Service of the U.S. Naval Hospital in Oakland, found a direct relationship between the amount of steroid metabolites in the urine and the severity of "clinical depressive symptomatology."[58] (The following year he tried, with considerable success, to treat "depressive reactions" with the steroid prednisone.[59]) In 1966, Robert Rubin and Arnold Mandell at the Neuropsychiatric Institute of UCLA summarized existing knowledge for readers of the *American Journal of Psychiatry*, concluding that "increased adrenal activity [is] a concomitant of psychological distress, depressive affect [is] a physiological reaction of the central nervous system to high circulating glucocorticoids," and that both depression and stimulation of the hypothalamic-pituitary-adrenocortical (HPA) axis were related to "a primary brain state alteration."[60] The endocrine system offered a window to the brain in psychiatry.

The National Institute of Mental Health (NIMH) and Walter Reed Hospital became important nuclei of research in neuroendocrinology. Many leaders in endocrine psychiatry got their start at one of these institutions. At Walter Reed, psychoanalyst David McKenzie Rioch established a neuroendocrine laboratory in the early 1950s, aided by David Hamburg, then at the hospital's Institute of Research. Rioch's co-workers included John Mason, Robert Rose, and Edward Sachar. As soon as Hamburg became chief of the Adult Psychiatry Branch of NIMH in December of 1957, he steered research in the neuroendocrine direction. Among his collaborators were James Maas, Francis Board, and John Davis.[61] Hamburg recalled their bewilderment in the mid-1950s, until the work of Geoffrey Harris (see above), about whether the hypothalamus could influence the pituitary. "There were just a few nerve fibrils connecting them; there was no rich nerve connection that could do the job. We did not realize until later that the job was done by chemical messengers."[62]

Indeed, early findings at NIMH and "The Reed" on the relation of the HPA axis and depression seemed counterintuitive because, as Hamburg said, "it was assumed at the time that a person sitting quietly, not communicating, and rather withdrawn and despondent would not have physiological or biochemical alarm responses, but that turned out not to be the case."[63]

In 1960, after training in psychiatry and psychoanalysis, William E. Bunney came to NIMH in the section on psychosomatic medicine. As "project chief for studies in biochemistry and behavioral factors in depressive reactions," Bunney and his co-workers in 1965, including Hamburg (by then in Stanford), probed the relationship between biochemistry and "psychotic depressive crises," finding that on the "crisis onset day," corticosteroids rose.[64] In 1965, Bunney and Jan Fawcett suggested an endocrine test for "suicide potential," concluding, "In some patients the psychic distress accompanying suicidal intent may be of such a quality and magnitude as to produce sustained changes in various endocrine subsystems. This may occur whether or not the distress is clinically evident."[65] In 1967, Bunney and Fawcett published an overview containing a definite note of excitement:

The findings of the studies thus far reviewed are in general agreement in the description of marked elevations of 17-OHCS [17-hydroxycorticosteroids; i.e., cortisol] in that group of depressed patients characterized by great distress, with features of anxiety and agitation. In these studies there is a positive correlation between the degree of elevation of various indices of adrenal function and independent ratings of depression for a high proportion of patients studied.[66]

This research marked a fundamental commitment of the NIMH to biological theories of mental illness. Two years later, in 1969, under the leadership of Martin Katz, chief of the Clinical Research Branch in NIMH's extramural division, the Institute held a milestone conference at the College of William and Mary in Williamsburg, Virginia, on "the psychobiology of the depressive illnesses," at which one of the five main sections was on endocrinology.[67]

Dexamethasone

Other investigators were examining cortisol in Cushing's disease, where the hormone is overproduced by the overstimulated adrenal gland. What happens to cortisol when Merck's artificial steroid dexamethasone is given to Cushing's patients?

Background: Administering an external steroid suppresses the adrenal cortex. Elevated steroid levels prompt the hypothalamus and pituitary to lower the secretion of their hormones—CRF, ACTH—thereby decreasing the secretions of the adrenal cortex. Normally, administering dexamethasone lowers the production of cortisol. (Subsequent research established that dexamethasone acts both on the pituitary and on the hypothalamus.[68]) But not in Cushing's disease: When given an external steroid, these patients maintain a high level of adrenal cortical output. In 1960, Grant Liddle, in the Department of Medicine at Vanderbilt University School of Medicine in Nashville, sought a method to suppress ACTH as a diagnostic test for Cushing's disease. He administered a 0.5-mg dose of dexamethasone every six hours for eight doses to 114 patients suspected of having Cushing's disease, plus a control group of hospital employees. Liddle was not the first researcher to give steroids in an attempt to differentiate ACTH-driven adrenal output from autonomous adrenal output, but, for technical reasons, he was the first to get it right. The patients whose high cortical output was pituitary driven stopped making cortisol when given dexamethasone. Patients whose high cortical output was due to Cushing's disease (i.e., an adrenal tumor) continued to make cortisol. They did not suppress cortisol secretion; they "resisted" suppression and could be labeled dexamethasone "non-suppressors."[69] (Liddle did not use this latter term.) If the dexamethasone suppression test worked in the diagnosis of Cushing's, would it work in other diseases? How about depressive mood disorders?

In 1966, the scene switched back to James Gibbons, who had moved to the department of psychological medicine at the University of Newcastle upon Tyne in the north of England. Did depressed patients have a different plasma cortisol response than controls, he and coauthor T. J. Fahy asked? No, the responses were the same, it was true merely that depressed patients had higher cortisol levels. After injecting 2 mg of dexamethasone, they took blood samples in twelve endogenously depressed patients and twelve controls at one, two, and three hours after injection (the investigators also had a baseline sample before the injection). The rate of decline in cortisol in both depressed patients and controls was identical.[70]

Yet technique is important, and in these early days no one knew the right one. Gibbons and Fahy sampled the blood after just three hours, which was much too soon. Subsequent research found that cortisol levels were higher later in the twenty-four-hour cycle. Thus, for a dose injected at 11:00 P.M., one might check at 4:00 P.M. the following afternoon. In any event, nonsuppression does indeed take place after an injection of dexamethasone. But the first time dexamethasone was tested, it struck out.

That same year, 1966, endocrinologist Peter Stokes at New York Hospital examined the dexamethasone test in psychiatric patients. The results were better. Like Liddle, he waited forty-eight hours before checking the blood cortisol. As Gibbons and McHugh had originally done, he used a chemical test (Peterson) that is specific for cortisol. Stokes found, "Our psychiatric patients did not suppress as normals with dexamethasone .... Twelve of the 16 patients did not suppress normally. Three did not suppress at all. The above data suggest that the usual negative feedback system for plasma cortisol regulation of ACTH secretion is chronically ineffective in some emotionally aroused patients."[71] (In these years it was not clear that the hypothalamus was involved, because CRH was not yet available for research purposes; hence the emphasis on ACTH, the pituitary hormone.)

But how about depression? Was the DST specific for depression, or did it just identify people who were "emotionally aroused"? In 1968, endocrinologist Michael Besser at St. Bartholomew's Hospital in London, together with P. W. P. Butler, administered dexamethasone over a forty-eight-hour period to three severely depressed patients. The three "resisted suppression," as the phrase was now used, meaning their cortisol values remained high after dexamethasone. After the depressive mood disorders were successfully treated with "a combination of elec-trotherapy and antidepressant drugs," these abnormalities disappeared. Word had it that several patients on this endocrinological unit had "pseudo-Cushing disease," with such symptoms as obesity, hyperten-sion, glucose intolerance, and mood changes, together with borderline-abnormal cortisol values.[72] As Bernard Carroll tells the story, "These patients were nonsuppressors to low-dose dexamethasone but not to high-dose dexamethasone. [Besser and colleagues] decided these patients did not have true Cushing disease. However, one or two of them turned up floating in the Thames. It was then that these endocri-nologists realized that cortisol values in depression were intermediate between true normal and true Cushing disease."[73]

Bernard Carroll is known to his friends as Barney. As these events were transpiring, he was on a path to making the dexamethasone suppression test famous as the first biological test in mood disorders.

4

Barney Carroll and Ed Sachar

It is not Laignel-Lavastine but Bernard Carroll and Edward Sachar who stand as the founders of modern endocrine psychiatry. Of vastly different backgrounds, they made their mark in very different ways. But at the end of the day, when the awards are handed out, they will be first in line; for Sachar, alas, it is too late.

Carroll

Barney Carroll was born in Sydney, Australia, in 1940. His father, who had left school in the ninth grade to support his widowed mother and four sisters, was the general manager of the Yellow Cab Company. Carroll grew up in Sydney, but for business reasons the family relocated to Melbourne, and in 1958, Carroll began undergraduate studies at the University of Melbourne, receiving a Bachelor of Science and an M.B. degree (Bachelor of Medicine, the equivalent of a North American M.D. degree) in 1964. As an undergraduate, in 1961 he spent a year of research in the laboratory of Sam Gershon, a pioneer in lithium treatment. In the Australian "summer" of 1961–1962, Carroll was a fellow in John Eccles' physiology laboratory at Australia National University in Canberra—it was Eccles who, when at Oxford, worked out the principle of synaptic transmission in the central nervous system. In Canberra, Carroll also worked with neurophysiologists David Curtis and Jeff

Watkins, who identified the neurotransmitter properties of glutamate, aspartate, and glycine.

While completing his clinical training between 1962 and 1964, Carroll said, in an unpublished memoir, "I maintained my contacts with the department of pharmacology, and I was thinking about a career in that area. The new antidepressant and antipsychotic drugs were hot topics of study in Melbourne at that time."

After receiving the M.B., Carroll started to study internal medicine at the Royal Melbourne Hospital. In 1966, as a second-year resident, he was exposed to endocrinology in a clinical rotation on F. I. R. ("Skip") Martin's service, learning about neuroendocrine function tests.

Carroll's memoir continues:

> Martin became my role model as a clinical investigator. In addition to my clinical duties, Skip set me to work on a research project dealing with hypothalamo-pituitary-adrenal (HPA) function tests. These were used on the endocrine service primarily to assess patients with diabetes mellitus who had undergone pituitary irradiation for treatment of retinopathy. In the course of that work I came to realize that HPA function tests could in principle provide a means to test the new neurotransmitter theories of depression and antidepressant drug action.

Later that year, Carroll rotated through Brian Davies' psychiatry service at the Royal Melbourne Hospital. "I began to discuss these ideas also with Brian Davies . . . [who had arrived in Melbourne as first chair of psychiatry in 1964]." Davies, said Carroll, "was already quite familiar with the early studies linking cortisol to mood change." Imipramine had been marketed in 1957 in Switzerland and followed quickly everywhere else. A review article by Alec Coppen, "Biochemistry of Affective Disorders" in 1967, had taken a careful look at monoamines and products of the adrenal cortex.[2] At this point Carroll decided to take up psychopharmacology and not to pursue internal medicine as a career.[3]

In 1967, Davies offered Carroll a specially created post in the department of psychiatry as "clinical supervisor." Carroll's job, in addition to seeing patients in Davies' outpatient clinic and rounding with him on the inpatient service, was "to develop a research program along the lines we had envisaged." Carroll began "to study a series of HPA function tests in depressed patients. It was necessary for me to learn the laboratory methods of measuring plasma and urinary cortisol determinations," for which members of the department of biochemistry proved helpful. "Through this process I first recognized the pattern of abnormalities in the dexamethasone suppression test (DST) associated with the clinical profile of endogenous depression or melancholia."

The first account of the DST "in patients with severe depressive illness" was published in the *British Medical Journal* in August of 1968 by Carroll, Martin, and Davies. In twenty-seven "typical melancholic patients" and twenty-two other patients with nondepressive illnesses, blood was sampled at 8:30 A.M. and 4:30 P.M. A 2-mg dose of dexamethasone was administered orally at midnight and then blood samples for estimation of plasma cortisol (11-OHSC) were taken the following day at 8:30 A.M. The pre-dexamethasone samples showed no differences between depressed patients and controls. The frequency distribution of the post-dexamethasone samples did. Also, at 4:30 P.M. the depressed patients had an average cortisol level of 15.1 micrograms per 100 cc of blood. After successful treatment, at discharge their cortisol levels had dropped to 9.4 micrograms per 100. The patients with the severest symptoms had the highest cortisol levels. Seventeen of the twenty-seven melancholic patients were treated with ECT, an indicator of the severity of their illness.[4] The report became a classic, referred to by over two hundred other researchers.

In the previous chapter we saw Gibbons and McHugh in the early 1960s establishing that depression was in part an endocrine disorder. When we asked Paul McHugh about Carroll's achievement, he said, "The thing about Barney Carroll was—that wonderful Australian—he saw what we had done, through his Australian chief, and he said, 'What Gibbons and McHugh did, that needs to be followed up on directly in relationship to diagnosis.' But [Edward] Sachar never did that. Carroll did that."[5] (Interestingly, Gibbons was not thrilled by Carroll's test. A few weeks after the article in the *British Medical Journal*, Gibbons, now at Newcastle, dismissed the results, saying the 2-mg dose had been far too high. The Australians must have "overridden" the negative feedback mechanism controlling cortisol, he said.[6])

After earning a doctorate degree in clinical psychobiology at Melbourne in 1971, Carroll left Australia for a two-year stint as clinical research fellow in the department of psychiatry of the University of Pennsylvania. His mentors in Australia now ceded senior authorship to him when publishing with Carroll in this area. From now on, the DST would be Carroll's affair.

Carroll had planned to return to Australia, but a shift in funding priorities of the New South Wales government left him at loose ends; in

1973 he took a post in the department of psychiatry of the University of Michigan in Ann Arbor. It was here in 1976 that he, together with John Greden and colleagues, established the Clinical Studies Unit for Affective Disorders (CSU). The CSU became an engine of clinical research.

What did the DST tell clinicians that simple cortisol levels did not? "If a system contains a fault," said Art Prange, a pioneer psychoendocrinologist at the University of North Carolina (UNC), "one is more likely to discover it by challenging the system rather than by passively observing it."[7] So rather than just observing differences in cortisol levels—which vary greatly from individual to individual—we will find out if the HPA axis itself is broken by challenging it with dexamethasone. Consider cortisol variation from patient to patient: At nighttime, for example, 65 percent of patients with melancholia have elevated cortisol levels, but so do 45 percent of patients with other diagnoses.[8] The feedback effect of the DST increases the "specificity" of a given cortisol reading. It standardizes the study of the endocrine system in depression by looking at the working of the HPA axis itself: Is it in order or not? Nonsuppression means it is not in order.

Over the next decade, Carroll established the principle of abnormal suppression of cortisol as the key feature of endocrine psychiatry. In melancholia, the hypothalamus hypersecreted CRF, stimulating the anterior pituitary, in turn activating the HPA axis and elevating serum cortisol levels. The HPA axis in melancholia does not respond to normal feedback signals to suppress the secretion of cortisol. Carroll revealed part of this powerful story; through determined publication and advocacy, he established the DST as a significant test of the endocrine system, even though he did not originate the concept. The DST was indeed, for better or worse, Barney Carroll's baby.

In his Melbourne doctoral research in 1972, Carroll reported that a positive DST did not result from the stress of illness, for schizophrenics and patients with other stressful illnesses did not exhibit abnormal DST responses.[9] Moreover, in 1976, Carroll, Joe Mendels at the Veterans Administration Hospital in Philadelphia, and George Curtis in Ann Arbor found that the cortisol disturbance in depression was subtler than in Cushing's disease. At 8:00 A.M., melancholic patients had normal levels of cortisol. Only later in the day did they "escape suppression" again (meaning cortisol was escaping the pituitary's suppression of the adrenal cortex and thus becoming elevated). They calculated that it was more rational to take post-dex samples within a twenty-four-hour cycle and not at 8:00 A.M. the following morning. This observation changed the ongoing procedures in a number of departments of psychiatry.[10]

In these early years, Carroll and co-workers suggested that the DST might be a useful laboratory test for melancholia (a distinct disorder often identified as endogenous depression and not just a synonym for severe depression). At the bedside, severity is not readily apparent, nor is it obvious whether suicide is being considered. A positive DST meant a melancholic depression, a red flare for high suicide risk. In 1976, Carroll wrote, "The dexamethasone suppression test may be of value as a laboratory aid in the diagnosis of 'endogenous' depression."[11] By 1977 it was clear that "[o]verall, about 40 percent of melancholic patients had abnormal DST results."[12] Indeed, given a tight definition of melancholia, virtually all melancholic patients—95 percent, he reported at a 1976 meeting in Strasbourg—had positive DSTs.[13] Carroll did not later insist on the 95 percent. But even a sensitivity of 50 percent was quite remarkable: melancholia was a homogeneous biological entity with a specific marker demonstrable in many patients (though not all) with a quantitative test.

What did melancholia look like in the clinic? The typical nonsuppressor, Carroll said, "resembles the classic melancholic clinical profile, has a high rate of recurrence and a strong family history, has a poor prognosis if the test does not normalize with drug treatment, and has the highest rate of specific response to antidepressant drugs." The physician should de-emphasize "psychosocial treatment" and be on guard for "violent suicide attempts."[14]

The implications of this work for the study of mood disorders were considerable. First, it meant that a clinician could tell with 50 percent certainty if the patient was melancholic and begin appropriate treatment: electroconvulsive therapy or tricyclic antidepressants were the best available.

Second, it offered a reliable measure of the risk of relapse. Patients with abnormal cortisol levels or who failed to normalize with dexamethasone were at greater risk of falling ill again than those whose cortisol levels had returned to normal.[15] Scoffers would later claim they did not need the DST because they believed they could tell clinically whether their patients had melancholia. But they could not tell clinically, in a group of apparently recovered patients, who was at risk of relapse and needed continued careful monitoring.

Finally, the research showed that there were two forms of depressive illness: One, which Carroll increasingly called "melancholia," had a biological base and called for somatic treatment (in those days psychotherapy alone was considered the principal treatment for psychiatric illnesses). The second depression—all the other forms of depressive moods—has since been termed "non-melancholia."[16] "The clinical differences between depressed patients who do and those who do not have increased cortisol secretion remain to be clarified," Carroll wrote in 1977. "It is possible that the two subgroups represent a fundamental heterogeneity within the depressive syndrome."[17] Three years later, in 1980, Carroll and a team from the CSU divided a population of depressed outpatients between those with endogenous depression (forty-seven) and non-endogenous (forty-six) on the basis of clinical characteristics, or "pattern recognition." Of the patients with endogenous depression, 40 percent had an abnormal DST; of the non-endogenous depressed, 2 percent had an abnormal DST. The DST, they said, thus had a sensitivity of 40 percent, a specificity* of 98 percent.[18]

Clearly, the Michigan team had not yet fully clarified the clinical characteristics of the DST nonsuppressors (the "positive" patients).

By the early 1980s, enough investigators had used the DST to make possible a comprehensive picture of the test and what it was able to spotlight. Of nine international studies, excluding Carroll's own, the sensitivity averaged 45 percent and the specificity 96 percent.[19] Carroll was later able to work out a gradient of DST abnormality in global severity of depression (using DSM-style diagnoses) that looks like this:[20]

Table 4.1 Severity of Depressive Illness and % Abnormal DST

Normal volunteers	~ 5%
Simple euphoric mania or hypomania	~ 5%
Bereaved persons	~ 7%
Minor depression or dysthymia	~ 15%
Bipolar II depression (major depression + hypomania)	~ 30%
Melancholic unipolar depression	~ 60%
Bipolar I depression (major depression + mania)	~ 60%
Bipolar I depression with psychosis	~ 75%
Mixed bipolar disorder	~ 85%

Such a gradient suggests that there may be biological groupings of the mood disorders running from everyday sadness and bereavement to severely ill melancholic patients who simultaneously demonstrate the

---

Sensitivity means how many patients who are positive for the disease are also positive for the test; *specificity* means how many false positives: those who are positive on the test but do not have the disease. The higher the sensitivity, the greater the chances of getting *all* the patients you are interested in; the higher the specificity, the greater the chances of including *only* those with the disease you are interested in.

symptoms of depression and mania. This is not necessarily a continuum, but a measure of the extent to which endocrine abnormalities are involved in the illness.

In 1981, Carroll wrote a widely noted (and, later, even more widely scorned) article in the *Archives of General Psychiatry* that made a tactical error in the title: "A Specific Laboratory Test for the Diagnosis of Melancholia," thus offering the procedure as a "screening test." Though Carroll did not actually use the term "screening test," it is the image of the DST that he offered when he wrote, "The routine use of this simple test by internists, family practitioners, and psychiatrists who treat depressed patients may help to reduce the diagnostic confusion we have described." (In the article, Carroll described patients with "non-endogenous" depression who were, in the practice of American medicine, treated inappropriately with lithium or tricyclic antidepressants.) Yes, he told doctors: the DST will end the puzzlement about mood disorders. This is how the article was perceived, even though Carroll said flatly that the DST was not "biologically specific" for melancholia, which was a weasel phrase, because earlier in the piece he had said that it was indeed "highly specific for melancholia."[21] At one point, Carroll did in fact recommend the DST for "screening."[22]

The 1981 article was a blunder. One enthusiastic psychiatrist said, "The article published in the *Archives of General Psychiatry* in 1981 was like a trumpet blast. It was everybody's dream to have a laboratory test, an objective indicator of the mental state in psychiatry."[23] One can see the problem already: such enthusiasm would create excessive and inappropriate use, followed by eventual disappointment. One source, who did not wish to be identified, said, "The title of the 1981 paper started the horse running in the wrong direction. People said, 'finally psychiatry is a part of medicine!'" Robert Rubin, a psychiatrist at the Veterans Administration Hospital in Los Angeles and long-standing researcher in neuroendocrinology, later said, "You need a pattern of suppression and escape to study the power of the HPA axis that is driving the abnormality." A single 4:00 P.M. test was a "disaster."[24]

Rather than going on to glory, the DST was about to come to an end.

What was Carroll's contribution to the endocrine psychiatry story? McHugh noted,

I thought Carroll's contribution was to focus on this elevated cortisol level. The measurement of steroids became steadily more easy. In the late 1950s, early '60s, it was a tough thing to do, I'm telling you! You had to work hard to get it. As it got easier, he began to follow up on the idea that not only was there an elevation in the morning—because it was always in the morning when he was doing it—he could show there was an elevation all day, and he began to think in terms of why it was. He began to think more physiologically, more coherently about what must be off, maybe a feedback loss, and follow up on that. I always thought that because both of us were trained, in a sense, in the Mayerian-Maudsley way [Willi Mayer-Gross], to really do a thorough, bottom-up examination, he could see that as a subgroup. Depression, he *knew* that depression was a symptom, but a subgroup of conditions could be identified perhaps in this physiological way, and he hammered away at that point, and I think that was his great contribution.[25]

Yet Carroll, a neuroscientist, did more than cobble together like a craftsman a useful tool. He sought a window to the brain, calling attention to dysfunction in the limbic system in particular as the source of melancholia, or, if not the sole source, an important stream of hormones pouring onto the illness. In 1980 he said that "[t]he several neuroendocrine disturbances...in endogenous depression, of which the abnormal DST response is...the most specific, may represent indirect functional markers of the associated disturbances in the limbic system. That is, they may be indicators of 'limbic system noise' with a temporal but epiphenomenal link to the primary pathology of the illness."[26] This is a powerful concept, but it has lain fallow since Carroll conceived it.

Sachar

In social terms, Edward Sachar had a quite different background than Carroll, coming from one of the great Jewish-American families and growing up in an atmosphere of intense intellectuality in St. Louis, where Edward's father, Abram Sachar, was a professor of history at Washington University. The theme of intellectuality in the Sachar family is recurrent: Abram himself was, according to Edward's brother David, the son of a merchant who had been "an outstanding student at his religious school in Poland." In 1948, Abram Sachar became the founding president of Brandeis University in Waltham, Massachusetts;

he wrote, among his other contributions, the one-volume Knopf classic *A History of the Jews* (1963), which has remained in print for more than forty years.

Said David, "For [our father's] three sons—Howard, Edward, and me—there was never any attraction to the world of business. While each of our professional pathways diverged in details, they were always within the boundaries of academia.... All three of us majored in history in college and maintained strong roots in the humanities throughout our lives."[27]

Edward's brothers went on to careers of distinction. Howard Sachar, born in 1928, became a well-known historian at George Washington University and author of the celebrated *History of the Jews in America* (1992); David Sachar, born in 1940, became director of gastroenterology at New York's Mount Sinai Hospital and an international expert on inflammatory bowel disease. Edward himself, the middle child, was born in 1933 and graduated with a bachelor's degree in history from Harvard College in 1952.

Why did Edward not become a historian, like his father and his brother? According to David,

Ed's decision to go to medical school was motivated, I believe, principally by the intention to enter psychiatry—a field that perhaps satisfied both the scientific instincts of his brain and the humanistic inclinations of his heart.... I remember his wide-eyed wonder when he first learned in a research lab that guinea pigs could be *conditioned* to have asthmatic attacks by a purely visual stimulus! His passion for probing the neurochemical and psychoendocrine mechanisms of psychiatric illness never abated from that day on.

Edward Sachar began medical studies at the University of Pennsylvania in 1952. He was turned on by research challenges after attending Marvin Stein's neuroendocrine lectures. Stein recalls, "I gave talks about stressing animals and measuring anti-diuretic substance and the effect of the adrenal and the effect of the hypothalamus.... Well, Ed got all excited, and came and said he wanted to work with me. So I said, 'well, we're working with guinea pigs now,' and he said, 'I'll work with you no matter what.' His job was to clean out the cages, so he cleaned out the guinea pig crap for the better part of a whole summer."[28] Sachar graduated in 1956 and interned in 1956–1957 at Beth Israel

Hospital in Boston, followed by a residency in psychiatry from 1957 to 1959 at the Massachusetts Mental Health Center, in the days when "Mass Mental" was given over largely to psychoanalysis. This was a potential pitfall.

Paul McHugh and Ed Sachar had known each other as medical students, McHugh at Harvard and Sachar at Penn. Both men were candidates for appointment as residents at Mass Mental: "We were exactly contemporaries as residents, and George Thorn [Harvard neurologist and physician-in-chief at the Brigham] said to me, 'don't go,' and I didn't go. Ed went. Ed went there, and he got enamored of Elvin Semrad [well-known psychotherapist at Mass Mental], while I was off on this *entirely* different trajectory."[29]

Thus, as we saw in Chapter 3, McHugh ended up training in psychiatry at the Maudsley while Ed Sachar was at Mass Mental. McHugh continued about the adventures of his friend Ed: "Elvin Semrad's idea about schizophrenia was that it was a stress-related breakdown, and he had crazy ideas about it. Ed got attracted to this, and he wanted to prove it with endocrines, and he started off in the direction of studying the schizophrenia cases, with their endocrines, at the very same time I was showing in the Maudsley that this [endocrines] worked with depression."

After Mass Mental, Sachar faced the question of military service during those years of the "doctors' draft." According to David Sachar, Edward had wanted a post at the National Institute of Mental Health as an officer in the Public Health Service, but his nearsightedness disqualified him. He therefore spent two years from 1959 to 1961 in the Army at the rank of captain at the Walter Reed Army Institute in the department of neuroendocrinology.

"The Reed" was an exciting experience for Sachar. In August of 1959, soon after arriving, he wrote to his parents, "My work setup is really superb—better than anything I could have imagined. I really should be paying them for the privilege of training with such splendid guys. It is without doubt going to be a wonderfully productive two years. They are so far ahead of anything else in this field—which I know! I'm a mighty lucky guy." (A young bachelor, he added, "The girls in Wash are really awful, that for every female college grad there are 10 male college grads + the Jewish girls are even scarcer.")[30]

According to McHugh, it was Ed Sachar who brought interest in endocrine depression to the NIMH in these years when Sachar was at the nearby Walter Reed Hospital. "Ed had persuaded Biff Bunney and a couple of other people at the NIH that endocrines were important, and they had re-discovered the idea of depression [and endocrines]. He at this time had started abandoning the Semrad concept of schizophrenia. It was crazy, that nutty idea."

From Walter Reed, Sachar got his first publication in 1961, together with John Mason and others at the hospital's Institute of Research, establishing the role of the limbic system in the secretion of ACTH.[31]

Edward returned to Beth Israel in September of 1961 for the final year of his residency, finishing in June of 1962. For three years he remained an associate in psychiatry at Harvard, while simultaneously undergoing training in psychoanalysis.

This was a tumultuous time in the social history of the United States. In August of 1964 Sachar worked with the Medical Committee for Human Rights, a group of New York physicians committed to social justice for black Americans in Mississippi, offering "emergency first aid to civil rights workers who were beaten, shot or otherwise injured." He later wrote, "I experienced the eerie sensation of becoming part of a newsreel," as he and a fellow physician "found a young white boy, covered with blood, cradled in the arms of a Negro worker who was trying to stop the bleeding."[32]

In 1966, Morton Reiser, who had organized a high-powered group of biological researchers in psychiatry at Montefiore Hospital in the Bronx, recruited Sachar for the department. Sachar became founding director of the psychoendocrine research laboratories; shortly thereafter he was appointed at the Albert Einstein College of Medicine, becoming professor of psychiatry in 1972 and chair of the department in 1975. Additionally, he was chief psychiatrist at the Bronx Municipal Hospital Center. Somewhat surprisingly for a biological psychiatrist, in 1972 he graduated from the New York Psychoanalytic Institute.[33]

Like so many American psychiatrists who trained in psychoanalysis in these years of perfervid interest in Freud—one of us (Fink) among them—Sachar soon abandoned psychoanalysis and turned to biology. Whereas Carroll had concentrated his work until the end of the 1980s upon a practical test, it was Sachar's ambition to gain a comprehensive picture of what happens to the endocrine system in depression or how the endocrine glands themselves cause and shape depression. Surrounded by enthusiastic acolytes, Sachar had made great progress in this direction when a stroke cut him down in 1980; he retired in 1981 and died by suicide in 1984.

The first dimension in Sachar's research in endocrine psychiatry involved the relationship between cortisol and the patient's psychological world: What psychic events govern the secretion of cortisol? One of Sachar's early papers, written in 1962 while at Walter Reed (he was a junior author together with David Hamburg), concerned psychological factors governing the excretion of 17-hydroxysteroids (having an OH group at position 17).[34] In these years, Sachar and his collaborators saw symptoms in psychoanalytic terms and bodily events in biochemical terms. In 1963, he viewed "acute schizophrenic reactions" as a function of "the effectiveness of the defenses, whether they be psychotic or neurotic."[35] It took a while for this jargon to fall away. In 1967, he and co-workers at the Psychoendocrine Research Laboratory and the Center for Clinical and Metabolic Studies of Affective Disorders of the Massachusetts Mental Health Center asked, How did psychotherapy influence corticoid secretion?[36] Also, how about "ego disintegration"?[37]

A second dimension, marked by deepening involvement in the late 1960s with other steroid researchers at Montefiore, entailed unpacking depression into the components that were apparently dependent on cortisol and those that were not. The biological components would later be called the "phenotype," or elements of illness thought to be genetically—or at least somatically—determined. Montefiore was a national center of steroid research, and Sachar's co-workers were all simultaneously professors at Albert Einstein College of Medicine, for which Montefiore Hospital was a clinical center. The team included Leon Hellman, chief of the hospital's Division of Neoplastic Medicine; Thomas Gallagher, a biochemist who was head of the hospital's Institute for Steroid Research; and David Fukushima, a co-worker at the Institute for Steroid Research. Gallagher and Fukushima were Ph.D.'s.

In 1969, Sachar's team went to the College of William and Mary in Williamsburg, Virginia, where, as we have seen, Martin Katz, chief of external clinical research at NIMH, had organized a conference on the biology of depression. To get a more precise measure of cortisol, the Sachar group had radiotagged external cortisol with an isotope, carbon 14; injected it; and then, free of the normal 17-hydroxycorticosteroid (17-OHCS) metabolites of cortisol, studied urinary cortisol output.[38] When they published the research in a psychiatry journal in 1970, the eleven patients on whom they reported in Williamsburg had increased to sixteen.[39]

The investigators found that cortisol levels rose significantly during illness only for some aspects of depression: mainly in the presence of psychosis (big increase) and anxiety (some increase). "In contrast, there was no correlation between cortisol production and scores for all other symptoms of depression."[40] Apathetic depressed patients showed no increase in cortisol. To be sure, some psychoanalytic jargon lingered on, relating cortisol to "more universal ego phenomena, such as the presence of neurotic 'signal' anxiety . . . ." Nonetheless, the research was an important first step in unpacking the biology of depression.

In 1972, the Sachar team reported on "cortisol production in mania."[41] In conjunction with Herbert Meltzer, then at the University of Chicago, in 1974 they established that serum prolactin was normal in schizophrenia (contrary to expectations of low prolactin to reflect elevated dopamine levels).[42]

The cortisol research accelerated a third dimension in Sachar's work: linking activity in the HPA axis to brain events. In these years, radioimmunassay (RIA) was just opening up the study of CRH, as well as the other hypothalamic peptides. These developments are discussed in Chapter 7, but one of Sachar's important contributions in 1971, together with oncologist Leon Hellman and pediatrician Jordan Finkelstein—all at Montefiore—involved injecting insulin into thirteen seriously depressed patients and then measuring the growth-hormone response with RIA. (The hypoglycemia produced by insulin acts as a provocative stimulus, sometimes termed a metabolic stress, to the HPA axis, as well as provoking growth-hormone release.) In five subjects, the GH response to hypoglycemia turned out to be "deficient"; the deficit lessened with recovery.[43] This study tested not the HPA axis but rather the hypothalamo-pituitary-somatotropic axis. Carroll had already demonstrated in 1969 that depressed patients have a blunted cortisol response to hypoglycemia and that this functional defect is associated with abnormal DST results.[44]

In 1973, Sachar and the other members of his steroid team, which now included internist Andrew Frantz (at Columbia), psychiatrist Norman Altman, and neurologist Jon Sassin (both at Montefiore), looked at the growth-hormone and prolactin responses in depressed patients to L-dopa and to hypoglycemia.[45] Plasma cortisol was measured every twenty minutes for twenty-four hours in six patients with psychotic depression and eight controls. The depressed patients secreted more cortisol. They had more secretory episodes, with more cortisol in each episode. Their adrenal cortexes were actively at work late at night and early in the morning, when the normal cortex is less active. After treatment with electroconvulsive therapy or imipramine, these patterns normalized. The authors found that "[t]he increased number of secretory episodes and time spent in active secretion would... reflect increased hypothalamic neuroendocrine activity presumably due to neural influences on the corticotrophin releasing hormone (CRH) secreting cells." In depression, they asked, could the receptors in the central nervous system for cortisol feedback-inhibition be less sensitive?[46]

This study of cortisol secretion and circadian rhythm was important for another reason as well. The 1960s had seen much psychodynamic reasoning about adrenocortical activation as the result of psychological defense mechanisms involving "failing defenses" and "ego disintegration." Sachar himself had shared these thoughts. Yet the discovery that nocturnal disinhibition, occurring partly in one's sleep, as a group of investigators at NIMH headed by David Rubinow pointed out, "was more difficult to reconcile with a psychological distress theory, as relative cortisol hypersecretion appeared even during sleep."[47]

Reaching out to internists, psychiatrists, and neurologists from Montefiore and Columbia, by 1973, the Sachar group set out to see how pituitary activity changes under alteration of brain events. They worked out the tactic of giving postmenopausal depressed women challenges of insulin on some occasions and L-dopa on others. The research is more remarkable for its conception than for what it actually demonstrated: A fall in plasma prolactin, for example, "would suggest that sufficient L-dopa had been converted to brain dopamine in these patients to induce the release of PIF [prolactin-inhibiting factor in the hypothalamus]."[48]

These were ingenious propositions, but there were too many variables, and the actual brain events that govern the endocrine system are far more complicated than was thought in 1973. Nonetheless, the investigators said, "We believe the data we have presented here support the evidence that there exists a central neurochemical disturbance (probably involving catecholamines [norepinephrine and dopamine]) in unipolar depressive illness."[49]

The Sachar group continued to explore brain–endocrine relationships. In 1975, they induced hypoglycemia in ten postmenopausal women with depression and in ten similar controls, observing the growth hormone response. (Normally, serum growth hormone would increase with hypoglycemia, but this response is blunted in depression.) Depressed patients increased their growth hormone by only 4.6 nanograms per milliliter and the controls by 13.3. "All of the normal subjects had clinically adequate HGH [human growth hormone] responses, in contrast to only four of the depressed patients." The blood glucose responses were the same (so there was no difference between depressed and controls in insulin action). The authors concluded: "Since brain catecholamines play a major role in mediating HGH responses to hypoglycemia, the findings are consistent with the hypothesis of diminished functional catecholaminergic activity in the depressed patients."[50] This was in line with the "catecholamine" theory of depression that Joseph Schildkraut had articulated in 1965—depression as a result of too little norepinephrine.[51] Robert Rose at the University of Texas Medical Branch in Galveston, who was another pioneering figure in endocrine psychiatry, said in 1984, "Ed Sachar...postulated maybe a decade ago the concept of a window on the hypothalamus."[52]

There is a gap between constructing suggestive hypotheses—as much of the above research did—and confirmation. Not all researchers were convinced that Sachar's neuroendocrine work confirmed the correctness of neurotransmitter theories of depression. Barney Carroll, for one, poured cold water on the enterprise at a meeting of the American Psychopathological Association that took place in March of 1975: "...The hypothesis suggested from the hypoglycemia study might appear to give experimental support to the general catecholamine theory of depression. This impression would be an unfortunate one.... The growth hormone system is an extremely complex one; it is by no means thoroughly understood, and at this stage clinical findings must be interpreted with caution."[53]

One final piece of work at Montefiore should be mentioned: Sachar's discovery that almost all antipsychotic drugs were effective in schizophrenia because they blocked dopamine activity and hence increased the secretion of prolactin. This finding was announced at the 1975 meeting of the American Psychopathological Association,[54] but was published as a definitive statement only in 1977, a year after Sachar decamped to the Psychiatric Institute, in a two-page note in the *Psychopharmacology Bulletin*.[55] Prolactin secretion thus represented a test of the clinical potency of antipsychotics, a test that is still widely used today.

In 1976, this productive period of research at Montefiore Hospital came to an end as Sachar accepted the chair of psychiatry at the New York State Psychiatric Institute of Columbia University. He had constructed a comprehensive picture of neuroendocrine aspects of depression, and the volume that he edited in 1976 of papers delivered the previous year at the American Psychopathological meeting devoted to hormones, behavior, and psychopathology represented a capstone to his life.[56]

At the New York State Psychiatric Institute (PI), Sachar's own work changed. In the four years between becoming chair and the stroke that ended his career in December of 1980, Sachar was able to do less hands-on research of his own but gathered about him a large and intellectually very active group of residents and junior staffers. One, Uriel Halbreich, later said that he was the only one who engaged in shouting arguments with Sachar.[57] But that you could shout at the chief and have your job the next day shows that the PI under Sachar was full of give-and-take.

A new theme at the PI was developing a rival to the dexamethasone suppression test, finding a new test with the same specificity (which was already close to 100 percent) but improved in sensitivity, the ability to identify all cases. Until then, the sensitivity of the DST was considered to be around 50 percent.

Sachar's work with amphetamine dated back at least to 1976 at Montefiore, when he, Robert Marantz, Elliot Weitzman, and Jon Sassin noted that amphetamine suppressed cortisol secretion in monkeys.[58]

In 1980, Sachar and his PI team—which included Greg Asnis, Swami Nathan, and Uri Halbreich—examined the impact of amphetamine on cortisol in humans. Halbreich was effectively in charge of this research. Giving depressed patients an injection of amphetamine in the morning produced a 33 percent drop in cortisol within ninety minutes. A control group showed no changes, maintaining high cortisol levels. When amphetamine was given to normal young men, it produced a *rise* in cortisol, "an acute response absent in ten of the 11 depressed patients." The authors speculated that amphetamine might "correct" a hypothetical brain "deficit" of norepinephrine.[59] The real significance of the finding did not strike them at once: They were looking at a biological measure of depression, an alternative to the DST.

This realization dawned the following year, in 1981. Injections of dextroamphetamine were given to twenty-two patients "with severe endogenous depressions" and eighteen normal controls. "While the normal subjects generally had a sharp increase in plasma cortisol level by 30 minutes after drug administration, two thirds of the depressed patients showed a paradoxical suppression of cortisol levels...." The authors thought this might serve as a "dextroamphetamine cortisol test" that warranted further study.[60]

In 1985 the Sachar group, minus its chief, who had died the previous year, proposed a d-amphetamine cortisol test (DACT). They detected 72 percent of "endogenous major depressive disorders," with a specificity of 88 percent—comparable to the DST—and a sensitivity of 72 percent, considerably higher than the DST. Further research was now needed, not compared to normals, the authors said, but to patients with other psychiatric illnesses.[61] This research was never done, and in the practice of psychiatry the DACT died (along with the DST).

The Sachar group sputtered along in the early 1980s, reporting that hypercortisolemia in endogenous depression is correlated with a shortened period from onset of sleep to the beginning of the rapid-eye-movement phase of sleep (called "REM period latency"). This added further strokes to the portrait of melancholia as a biological illness.[62] But the life went out of endocrine psychiatry at the Institute. Sidney Malitz became acting director in December of 1980. In 1984, Herbert Pardes became the new director of PI, taking the research of the Institute in other directions.

It was in 1979, just before the events that had such a fateful impact on endocrine psychiatry, that Edward Sachar summed up the promise of the research he had been guiding: "The rapid development of this field in less than two decades permits optimism that major depressive illness will be among the first 'functional' psychiatric disorders to have its chemical pathology elucidated."[63]

What was Ed Sachar's contribution? When McHugh returned from England, he and Sachar had a heart-to-heart.

McHugh: I would tell him I thought that the Elvin Semrad stuff was off the wall, and he gradually began emphasizing the fact that more and more studies should be done with human beings in endocrine . . . . He stimulated a lot of good people to become interested in neuroendocrinology. He did much more than I ever did in getting people to do that.

Interviewer: Sachar's role in neuroendocrinology?

McHugh: I think his only role was to show that there was gold in them thar hills.

Interviewer: And attract others to it?

McHugh: And attract other people. He was a very attractive person.[64]

5

The DST in Use

In February of 2006, the current authors were having a conversation with psychiatrist Walter Brown, who in the early 1980s was associate chief of staff at the Veterans Administration Medical Center in Providence, Rhode Island.

Fink told Brown the paper that got him first interested in the DST was Barney Carroll's contribution to the Mowbray and Davis volume in 1972.[1] For Fink, the immediate stimulus was the meeting of the American Psychopathological Association in 1975, where Ed Sachar gave an overview of his own endocrine research and edited the proceedings that came out the following year.[2] Brown agreed those were the landmark events for him as well. In 1976, Fink received a consulting appointment at a Veterans Administration Hospital on Long Island. The conversation continued:

Fink: I had a fellow at that time, Yiannis Papakostas, who had come from Athens and worked with me first as a resident [at Stony Brook], and then moved to our unit at the VA at Northport. He was the attending psychiatrist on the unit, and I was the consultant from the university. And I would come there every morning. We found that to separate depression as we understood it—which was really *DSM-II* manic-depressive illness– from schizophrenia was not easy.... We had the "pure" [psychotics]—but they were far from an easy diagnostic problem. And so we had some problems with doing the [dexamethasone suppression] test in terms of separating what we called depression [from schizophrenia]. The test was proposed first as a measure of illness, not as a test of depression. Sachar, Carroll, other writers at the time said, "If you happen to be severely enough depressed to be referred for ECT"—that's Sachar's statement— "you have a very high index of abnormal cortisol. And especially it goes in a diurnal cycle, and then when you give a steroid, it doesn't suppress." Confirming Carroll and Mowbray and that sort of thing. And we accepted that. From the ECT world. It became a critical variable. It was of great interest to us that also—after the patient got better with ECT—this test changed.

Walter Brown: Yup.

Fink: Plus one other thing. When my patients . . . relapsed, I found that the normality became abnormal again.

Brown: Yeah, we saw that, too.

Fink: Papakostas and I confirmed that our ECT patients did beautifully in reversing the abnormal DST. And when one or two of them got sick again—which they did, ECT was stopped prematurely in those days—the abnormality came back.[3]

Many clinicians of that generation found the DST a reliable gauge of whether patients had a melancholic illness, not whether they were sick, and of telling when they had finally recovered. In the 1970s and 1980s, it spread throughout psychiatry.

Dissecting Depression

The experienced physician does not need the DST to tell if the patient is seriously ill. But there must be something clinically distinctive about these patients who, compared to all others who are depressed, seem to have a common biology. They have distinctive markings. What are they? The DST flourished because it aroused the curiosity of a generation of scientifically inquisitive psychiatrists.

In the early 1980s, George Arana was a resident in psychiatry at McLean Hospital near Boston. The residents routinely ordered DSTs, as he later said in an interview:

[We used it in] anybody in whom you had a question about the diagnosis of depression, where you wanted to get guidance on, "Do I treat with an antidepressant, do I treat with an antidepressant and an antipsychotic, do I treat with an antipsychotic first and just wait and see what happens?" In that situation, when you're trying to make a differential diagnosis, if you do the DST and it's positive, you'd charge ahead with the antidepressant and you're thinking affective illness.... And it was a routine test that we would order.[4]

Awareness soon dawned that the DST was not a quantitative measure of severity but a qualitative measure of kind. As Robert Rose at the University of Texas Medical Branch in Galveston said in 1983,

One of the things that is perplexing about the dexamethasone test is that there is no continuum of response. The more seriously ill patients do not show more profound impairment of dexamethasone suppression and there is no correlation with the Hamilton [depression] scores, for example. Why is it that among those who do escape suppression, there is no relationship between the magnitude of illness and magnitude of cortisol abnormality?[5]

(It is possible that within melancholia, the DST does measure severity, but it is not a measure of the severity of "major depression" as defined by *DSM* criteria.)

Among the many varieties of depressive illness, what type did it spotlight?

Was it the primary-secondary typology associated with George Winokur and the St. Louis school, later at the University of Iowa when Winokur became chair there? Largely abandoned today, the typology distinguished between primary and secondary unipolar affective disorders ("primary" meant depression in someone without any other psychiatric diagnosis; "secondary" meant depression in a person with a "preexisting nonaffective primary psychiatric disorder"). The primary was subdivided into bipolar and unipolar; the primary unipolar then subdivided into familial pure depression, sporadic depression, and depression spectrum. In 1980, Winokur and co-workers reported that 44 percent of the primary unipolar depressives and none of the secondary unipolars were DST nonsuppressors. There was also clear differentiation among those with familial pure depressive disease (76 percent nonsuppressors), sporadic depressives (44 percent) and depression-spectrum patients (7 percent). It was unclear what this meant, save that a family history contributed strongly to a positive DST. The most impressive results were for bipolar depression: 85 percent were nonsuppressors (none of the manic patients were nonsuppressors).[6]

The highest nonsuppression scores were often found among patients in mixed manic-depressive states. Of the seven patients with mixed type bipolar disorder whom Dwight Evans and Charles Nemeroff at the UNC tested in 1983, all were nonsuppressors.[7]

The DST had positive results in "masked depression," meaning endogenous depressive illness overlaid with the somatic complaints of pain and paresthesias. Zoltàn Rihmer and Mihàly Aratò in Budapest reported that, of sixteen female patients with masked depression, twelve exhibited an abnormal DST. "These results suggest that masked depression is a special form of primary (endogenous) depressive illness," they concluded.[8]

How about melancholia, often called "endogenous depression"? In these patients, the DST nonsuppression scores were very high. The biological abnormality the DST spotlights occurs preferentially in patients with melancholia. In 1986, the Hungarian group found that 57 percent of their female inpatients with melancholia had an abnormality of either the DST or the thyroid-stimulating hormone (TSH) (versus 14 percent of the nondepressed inpatients).[9] In 1986 William Coryell at the University of Iowa captured the conviction of many authors of DST studies "that the DST effectively distinguishes between two groups of depressed patients whose features are consistent with the theoretical predictions surrounding the concepts of endogenous and neurotic/reactive depression." Researchers did not believe a counter-literature that questioned the specificity of the DST: such findings were more a result of "diagnostic heterogeneity [read 'poor diagnosis'] than DST nonspecificity."[10]

Is "endogenous depression" the biological entity the DST identifies? Surely there must be more to the story than that, because Carroll thought he was studying endogenous depression and found a sensitivity of only 50 percent. Why did the other half of the endogenous depressives not have a positive DST? In 1987 two groups of researchers characterized DST responders much more precisely. Dwight Evans and Charles Nemeroff at the UNC found the percent of DST nonsuppression (plasma cortisol of 5 micrograms per deciliters and above) as follows:[11]

Table 5.1 Rates of Dexamethasone Nonsuppression in Psychiatric Patients

Mixed bipolar	100%
Major depression with psychosis	95%
Major depression without melancholia	48%

Something about the admixture of psychosis and affective disorder increased nonsuppression markedly, especially in patients with mixed states.

In 1987, Kevin Miller and Craig Nelson at Yale undertook a factor analysis using the Yale Depression Inventory of symptoms associated with nonsuppression. They found the strongest associations with agitation, initial insomnia, loss of sexual interest, and weight loss. These intensely biological symptoms are commonly called "vegetative symptoms of depression." Psychological symptoms such as paranoia, guilt, feelings of worthlessness and helplessness were rarely associated with DST abnormality. While this finding goes back to the earliest days of HPA axis research, it is nonetheless interesting to see it confirmed. The authors noted that their DST nonsuppressors did not have some of the classic symptoms of endogenous depression, such as loss of interest, anhedonia, or "lack of reactivity."[12] So, clearly, the DST was picking up a biological dimension of melancholia, rather than a mental or psychological dimension.

Clinicians would know that the psychotic patients, loaded with vegetative symptoms and in the grip of mixed mania-melancholia, were ill and needed to be treated; they did not need the DST to tell them that. But what biological processes in these patients produce these alarming symptoms?

Fine-Tuning

The DST never had a chance to be fine-tuned. It disappeared before the basic questions that might be asked of any test were answered. But at least the fine-tuning began.

How about the dose, 1 mg or 2 mg? In 1985 Walter Brown made a strong case for the 2-mg dose. Vexed with problems in specificity—the DST's turning positive for many nondepressed patients and for normal individuals—Brown and co-workers set out to see if the dose was too low. They compared urinary cortisol levels in patients receiving 1- and 2-mg doses: "With the common 1-mg DST, 24-hour urinary cortisol levels in nonsuppressors and suppressors did not differ. With the 2-mg DST, however, nonsuppressors had significantly higher urinary cortisol levels than suppressors." Thus, the 1-mg dose was inadequate to identify those patients with a disturbed HPA axis. Only with the 2-mg dose did nonsuppressors reliably have higher cortisol.[13]

These reports caused a brief flurry of excitement among DST defenders at a time when the test was increasingly coming under attack as irrelevant to clinical psychiatry. In February of 1985, just after Brown's article appeared, John Worthington, medical director of Huntington Hospital in Willow Grove, Pennsylvania, wrote to Brown, "It was very enheartening to read this article since so much of the DST literature recently has been disappointing and I was begrudgingly having to believe it. My thought now is that with this dosage change, we can salvage the test and still get some pragmatic help from it."[14] Brown later said regretfully that the DST was repudiated because of an artifact: the use of the 1-mg dose. "But a 2-mg DST may be a more valid indicator of pituitary-adrenocortical hyperfunction; the results of a 1-mg DST may be more vulnerable to extraneous influences . . . . Unfortunately, before these procedural matters could be sorted out, the DST was repudiated."[15]

But let's not get ahead of our story.

The specificity question appeared crucial. What other diseases elicited an abnormal DST? Will all the cases it picks up be reliably the same disorder, or will wild cards be included? As early as 1969, it became apparent that other conditions in psychiatry also caused nonsuppression. In 1969, V. H. Asfeldt, an internist at Steno Memorial Hospital in Gentofte, Denmark, trying to fine-tune the 1-mg DST as a screening test for Cushing's disease, noted nonsuppression in patients with obesity, anorexia nervosa, juvenile diabetes, and epileptics on anticonvulsants, who were unlikely to have Cushing's disease.[16] He did not look at depressed patients. This was an early warning that the DST was sensitive to starvation and the effects of medications.

But there are virtually no tests in medicine with perfect sensitivity and specificity, so this was not necessarily a reason for rejection. The electrocardiogram, for example, "detects only around 50 percent of life-threatening AMIs [acute myocardial infarctions, heart attacks] in patients admitted with chest pain," as N. Herring and D. J. Paterson at the Burdon Sanderson Cardiac Science Centre at Oxford reported in 2006.[17] Yet we do not reject the electrocardiogram (ECG). The positive predictive value of magnetic resonance imaging for detecting unrecognized breast cancer in the second breast is, according to a study at the University of Washington Medical Center in Seattle, 21 percent overall and as low as 11 percent in premenopausal women.[18] In patients with unquestioned epilepsy, single electroencephalogram records are abnormal in only 56 percent.[19] Yet neurologists would not discard EEGs on the grounds that they are "insufficiently sensitive."

We must therefore be careful not to hold the DST to unrealistic standards. These biological markers are not specific tests of illness severity but rather markers of some brain disturbance, a note that something is wrong rather than a thermometer of distress. Carroll said in 1984,

> It is important to underline that whatever this test is telling us, it is only indirect information about some disturbance in the limbic system. It is not directly linked to the etiology of the psychiatric disorder, and is only an indirect indicator. This explains the lack of relationship to severity—a little like having EEG recordings where the severity of the electrical disturbance does not really correlate with the severity of the behavioural disorder, such as in limbic epilepsy.[20]

What about sensitivity and specificity in the DST?

In 1975 Peter Stokes and collaborators analyzed DSTs in consecutive admissions to the Payne Whitney Clinic, the psychiatry service of the New York Hospital–Cornell Medical Center. They gave a 1-mg dose at 11:00 P.M. and drew blood samples at 9:00 A.M. the following morning. They reported that 46 percent of the depressed group, 17 percent of the schizophrenic group, and 25 percent of other patients resisted cortisol suppression. According to these data, the DST was anything but specific for depression; rather, it was mildly suggestive. But the blood samples were taken at the wrong time, and over a twenty-four-hour cycle the results might have been different.[21] These data were, however, later thrown in the face of DST supporters.

Some studies found high DST sensitivity; others reported much lower sensitivities. At the Veterans Administration Hospital in Manhattan, a team led by Eric Peselow compared blood samples taken at 8:00 A.M. and 4:00 P.M. the following day. The sensitivity for depression of the 8:00 A.M. samples was 54 percent; for the 4:00 P.M. samples it was 92 percent.[22] Not bad. On the other hand, Ru-Band Lu and collaborators studied DSTs over a twenty-four-hour cycle in the psychiatric service of a teaching hospital in Taipei. They found the sensitivity of the DST in melancholia was only 63 percent, the same as in the depressed phase of bipolar illness; "schizophrenia with depression" was 43 percent; dysthymic disorder (*DSM-III*'s term for chronic depression), 12 percent; and normal volunteers, 10 percent.[23] For those who believed the DST would detect virtually all cases of melancholic illness, these were disappointing outcomes.

What could possibly account for such variable results? There were several circumstances. For one thing, different patients evidently metabolized dexamethasone at different speeds. Ross Baldessarini, a neuropsychopharmacologist at McLean Hospital in Belmont, Massachusetts, and George Arana, at the Boston VA Medical Center, discovered in 1984 that patients with "high concentrations of cortisol (positive DST) had 3.84 times *less* dexamethasone than those with negative DST results." Clearly, there was an inverse relationship between the amount of dexamethasone in the blood and nonsuppression: patients who metabolized quickly would show much more nonsuppression than those who metabolized slowly. The authors considered these rather paradoxical findings to bring the very validity of the DST into question: "These results suggest that a positive DST (nonsuppression of cortisol) in some psychiatric patients may reflect altered bioavailability of pharmacokinetics of dexamethasone, rather than a defect in the limbic-hypothalamic-pituitary-adrenal axis that results in overproduction of cortisol." At the very least, said the authors, DSTs should be accompanied by assays of serum dexamethasone itself, "to ensure that the level of exogenous steroid attained is sufficient to suppress cortisol production."[24]

This Baldessarini finding could be considered either fine-tuning or the first step in discarding the DST. Unfortunately, before the finding could be explored, the DST was clinically rejected.

The Manual

A bit of background: There had been growing uneasiness in psychiatry about the validity of the psychiatric diagnoses in vogue in the 1960s and 1970s. How reliable were the criteria for "depression," "primary and secondary," and "endogenous and reactive"? The criteria embedded in *DSM-II* were inadequate and unreliable. A major challenge to the "schizophrenia" diagnosis arose in 1971 in the U.S.–U.K. studies, which found "schizophrenia" to be much commoner in the United States than in the United Kingdom. ("Patient E," for example, was diagnosed as "schizophrenic" by 85 percent of American psychiatrists, but by only 7 percent of British psychiatrists.)[25]

This discontent gave rise to several attempts to improve the classification of psychiatric illness. Among the earliest was George Winokur and Paula Clayton's effort to separate bipolar from unipolar depression in 1967 on the basis of genetic and clinical factors.[26] Both investigators came from the "St. Louis School," meaning the department of psychiatry at Washington University in St. Louis. In 1970, Eli Robins and Samuel Guze, among the principal members of the St. Louis School, proposed a "method for achieving diagnostic validity" that followed the medical model of diagnosis—careful description of clinical signs and course, laboratory tests, follow-up results, and family-history information.[27] Richard Abrams and Michael Alan Taylor, then at the State University of New York at Stony Brook, suggested in 1976 that, on the basis of given motor signs, catatonia might be included in the circle of official diagnoses.[28] And in 1975, a task force of members of the St. Louis School and the New York State Psychiatric Institute took a first swipe at the comprehensive reevaluation of the whole system of psychiatric diagnoses.[29] So in the world of diagnosis-building there was lots of ferment.

These efforts were all part of the effervescence that led to a general reworking of psychiatric diagnoses in 1980, although most of these research-based diagnoses did not actually make it into this new guide, but served mainly to set the leaves rustling in the woods.

The third edition of the *DSM* series in 1980 did incorporate one revision of considerable significance for the dexamethasone suppression test: What had been considered a single manic-depressive illness underwent a large historic alteration.

The story is this: In 1980 the Task Force on Nomenclature and Statistics of the APA introduced a new classification of psychiatric disorders called *The Diagnostic and Statistical Manual of Mental Disorders, Third Edition*, or *DSM-III* (the first edition appeared in 1952). Led by Robert Spitzer, a psychoanalytically trained biometrician at the New York State Psychiatric Institute, the new *Manual* introduced the concept of "major depression" instead of the previous mood diagnoses of "manic depressive illness" and "depressive neurosis" of *DSM-II* (1968).[30] The previous edition had distinguished clearly between serious and not-so-serious depressions, but *DSM-III* conflated the two, because dysthymia, the other depressive diagnosis in *DSM-III*, was more a measure of chronicity than severity. For a single episode of depression, *DSM-III* would have only one diagnosis: major depression.[31] The change also divided depression in to unipolar depression (in major depressive disorder) and bipolar depression (in bipolar disorder). These huge historic changes merged endogenous depression and non-endogenous depression (and even though *DSM-III* included a "melancholic subtype" for major depression, it was really only a pale shadow of melancholia).

Major depression thus seized the imagination of the field in the way that whiplash had once done: James R. Hodge described in 1971 supposed whiplash injuries of the neck following auto accidents as a concept: "Magnificent in its simplicity and how it seizes the imagination of patients, doctors and lawyers."[32] This hypnotic simplicity, said Gordon Parker, head of the Black Dog Institute in Sydney, Australia, and pioneer of the distinction between melancholia and non-melancholia as the principal mood disorders, is what "major depression" possessed, a "concept, initially understandable and even admirable, [that] has accrued entity status and explanatory properties beyond its station." Parker said that "its transubstantiation to 'entity' status has led to conceptual confusion and to sterility in both depression research and clinical management."[33]

The basic problem with *DSM-III* was that the diagnoses were constructed solely on the basis of phenomenology, a checklist of signs and symptoms of the current illness, rather than using family history, response to treatment, past psychiatric history, and biological markers to limn disease entities.

One of us (Fink) noted this in 1978 when a draft of *DSM-III* was being circulated for comment. Fink mentioned how an ECG might change a diagnosis of "neurotic behavior" that had been based solely on what the patient seemed to have (phenomenology). "By excluding laboratory data and response to stimuli in the classification, I think you are artificially limiting the clues available to the psychiatrist, and indicating that the only thing the psychiatrist should do is talk, listen, write, and interview. In recent psychiatry the importance of laboratory data has been emphasized, and we should encourage psychiatrists in their classification and practice to use laboratory tools even if they are imprecise at present."

Spitzer was in the audience and replied, "I do not believe that any laboratory tests currently available can be used in a way that is comparable to their use in the rest of medicine. For that reason I think it would be premature and not useful to include laboratory procedures as part of the operational criteria for making a diagnosis in *DSM-III*."[34]

This disagreement between Fink and Spitzer was so fundamental as to constitute two separate views of the psychiatric enterprise. But it certainly produced different outlooks on the DST.

In an interview in 2007, Spitzer expressed surprise at the notion that the *DSM* might have been partly responsible for the death of the DST. "Really? How so? By not recognizing melancholia?" he asked.

Shorter responded, "The DST scores for major depression are pretty low. DST scores for melancholia are very high."

Spitzer then listened in silence as Fink made in the interview the same argument that Spitzer had rejected out of hand in 1975:

You [the *DSM* drafters] didn't adopt any laboratory tests because they weren't very valid. I think if one is to look back at what we have learned since the 1970s, there are a number of tests which have become a model. The lactate infusion is a model for defining a population.[35] If you really want to know if people have panic disorder, go one step further. You don't do it on everybody, you don't have to do it clinically, but certainly you should do it if you want to define a population—especially, for example, if you want to look for genes.

Thus, Fink averred, the utility of these biological tests such as the DST was not in screening or confirming what one could learn clinically anyway. It was as a research tool in specifying what clinical characteristics people have in common who are positive for the DST, or the lactate-infusion test in panic, or any of several other biological tests now available in psychiatry.

Spitzer listened attentively as Fink made this point, then changed the subject.[36]

With *DSM-III's* major depression, both the sensitivity and the specificity of the DST sank. Paul McHugh later said, "You see, Baldessarini is perfectly right, the DST does not fit *DSM* major depression. It's not because DST is not specific, it's because *DSM* is not specific enough."[37]

Carroll, furious that this new artifact of major depression was being used to validate the DST, told the American Psychopathological Association at its annual meeting in 1988, "No external validator can do better than the diagnostic system against which it is being compared.... As long as the validation is limited to a comparison of external laboratory measures against clinical features, it is impossible to make any progress, and it is very likely that type 2 errors [missing a real difference] can be introduced."[38] On another occasion, Carroll said of the *DSM*, "This change had the effect of creating a nonvalidated 'gold standard' against which the DST was inevitably compared."[39] The DST had been developed on the basis of criteria in the *International Classification of Diseases* (ICD) of the World Health Organization, the most recent of which in the years that the DST was winning acceptance was adopted in 1975.[39] Now it was to be validated on the basis of quite different criteria that cut Nature less precisely at the joints.

Carroll looked back with some unhappiness on the behavior of the leaders of psychiatry when *DSM-III* was released in 1980:

Carroll : When *DSM* came out, with their hand on their hearts, "We all have to remember," they solemnly said, "the *DSM-III* criteria are only hypotheses that need to be tested." And having said that, they persuaded a lot of people to swallow it—and once they got it through, they proceeded to act authoritarian rather than scientific, and not to allow any questions.

Interviewer : So it became carved in stone?

Carroll : And that's essentially why the DST ran up against *DSM*.

Interviewer : So *DSM* vanquished the DST?

Carroll : Yes.

Interviewer : Because it lost its specificity?

Carroll : Yes.

Interviewer : That's the story in a nutshell.[41]

Being used to measure a *DSM*-created artifact, the validity of the DST sank. In an analysis in 1989 of sixty-six inpatients "with a clear depressive syndrome," Carroll found that the *sensitivity* of the DST in *ICD-9* was 45 percent and in *DSM-III*, 35 percent; the *specificity* in *ICD-9* was 96 percent and in *DSM-III* 73 percent.[42] Few clinicians were aware of the differences between *ICD-9* and *DSM-III* in terms of dexamethasone test results. Yet, as the 1980s wore on and more and more DST results based on the *DSM-III* classification came in, disbelief grew (see Chapter 6).

Carroll's observation that *DSM-III* killed the DST seems accurate. Confronted with measuring an entity that was very poorly defined, the test performed ever more poorly, causing a loss of confidence in a profession prone to herd behavior. And suddenly the herd surged away from a procedure that had once shone so brightly.

What Remained?

If in fact psychiatrists were able to discern clinically whether they were dealing with a serious depression that required pharmacotherapy or ECT, what reason remained for using the DST?

For one thing, DST nonsuppressors were much more likely to make a serious suicide attempt; indeed, they were more likely to complete suicide. In a five-year follow-up study in 1990 of seventy-six inpatients with major depression at the University of Iowa, William Coryell established that "non-suppressors were nearly three times more likely to make psychologically serious suicide attempts during follow-up."[43] Returning to this theme again in 2001 at a fifteen-year follow-up, Coryell discovered that "the estimated risk for eventual suicide in this group [of nonsuppressors] was 26.8 percent, compared to only 2.9 percent among patients who had normal DST results."[44] In other words, nonsuppressors had a risk of completing suicide ten times as high as that of suppressors. This is certainly worth knowing in one's patients. (A decade later, this finding was confirmed.[45])

By extension, the DST can also identify patients who have not really recovered clinically (despite appearances to the contrary) and who may not stay well after treatment. Ivan Goldberg at the New York Psychopharmacologic Institute first discovered this in February of 1980, using a "modified" DST (administering dexamethasone at 11:00 P.M. on the first day, then drawing a blood sample at 9:00 A.M. on the third day [34 hours later]): "Of 5 suppressors on this second DST none relapsed within two months while all 3 non-suppressors had a return of depressive symptoms." (He saw it as an indication of when antidepressant therapy might be safely stopped).[46]

John Greden at the University of Michigan confirmed this later in 1980, comparing ten depressives whose abnormal DSTs at admission had become normal at discharge with four whose DSTs had failed to convert at discharge. "On all measures, those whose DST failed to convert showed substantially less improvement.... Use of the DST prior to discharge may help discriminate between patients whose remaining symptoms reflect situational or psychosocial problems and those with a continuing endogenomorphic process."[47] In a meta-analysis in 1993 of 144 articles on the relationship between DST and treatment response, Saulo Ribeiro and his colleagues at the University of Michigan found that *baseline* nonsuppression did not predict course after discharge. The important finding was that "persistent nonsuppression of cortisol on the DST *after* treatment was associated with high risk of early relapse and poor outcome after discharge."[48] So, if one's patients still have positive DSTs on discharge, they are not well, whatever their apparent clinical status. Treatment must be continued. This is important information.

Third, DST results give some indication of treatments to avoid as well as which to choose. In 1985, Walter Brown discovered that nonsuppressors have virtually no placebo response: 59 percent of suppressors responded to placebo compared to 8 percent of nonsuppressors.[49] This finding was soon confirmed.[50] Carroll commented on it much later:

> The most important conclusion I emphasized from these data is that DST-positive cases must not be assigned to treatment with CBT [Cognitive Behavioral Therapy] or IPT [Interpersonal Psychotherapy] or simple counseling. For them use of drugs or ECT is mandatory. This therapeutic guideline was especially salient in clinical settings like community mental health centers where most of the assessment and the treatment is done by non-psychiatrists.... I had many occasions when a psychiatrist working in the public mental health sector thanked me for introducing the DST, because it enabled them to get patients onto the right track with treatment.[51]

The few studies of psychotherapies in DST suppressors and non-suppressors show that psychotherapy does not work for the nonsuppressors, confirming Carroll's claim.[52]

As for medication, there have been no formal clinical trials. But it is widely agreed among experienced clinicians that in dexamethasone nonsuppressors, one would use tricyclic antidepressants and not SSRIs.[51] There are hints of differential responsiveness to noradrenergic drugs in nonsuppressors. In 1985 a group at the National Institute for Nervous and Mental Diseases in Budapest argued that DST nonsup-pressors did better on noradrenergic drugs such as maprotiline than on (what were in their view) serotonergic agents, such as amitriptyline.[54] Three years later, in 1988, Walter Brown summed up the scant litera-ture on specific treatment: "Whereas nonsuppressors appear to respond well to desipramine and imipramine, they show a poor response to clomipramine and mianserin." Suppressors, in contrast, did equally well on all these agents.[55] With the virtual disappearance of the DST, there have been few further treatment studies, but these suggestions are interesting. Surely, the treatment algorithm for post-discharge planning can only be strengthened by knowledge of the resolution of cerebral abnormality.

The DST also predicted which patients with psychosis would recover. William Coryell found that those with high postdexamethasone cortisol tended to recover within a year.[56] The implication was that those without an HPA abnormality would need extended treatment. Thus, a negative DST result, or suppression, might suggest treating a "schizoaffective disorder" patient with something other than an anti-depressant early on.

Finally, DST abnormalities predict which patients will respond well to electroconvulsive therapy.[57] Given that nonsuppressors are often among the sickest patients, it is immensely gratifying to the family, and enormously therapeutic, to be able to say that a patient right now curled into a fetal ball or pacing the wards, crying, "It's all my fault, it's all my fault," will next Friday night probably be able to go out for pizza with the family. Indeed, a positive dexamethasone test may well be an inducement to the family to consent to ECT. These are not trivial benefits.

"Look, it needs to be done!" said Paul McHugh in an interview.

Carroll really found something. And I have used it from time to time, and it has been a tremendous help to me in . . . difficult cases. People would say, "no, he doesn't have an affective disorder," and I would say, "no, this guy's got melancholia, you don't realize it," and we'd do it and it would come back, and with the DST then I could persuade people to get ECT and then they'd get better.[58]

The failure of the DST in the 1980s to gain traction in the face of these encouraging results frustrated many scientists and clinicians. Yet, in the world of research, the usefulness of the DST in delineating different kinds of depressive illness continued to be confirmed. In 1982, John Rush at the University of Texas Southwestern Medical Center in Dallas firmly advocated the existence of a kind of biological depression contrasted with a nonbiological one—"endogenous" vs. "non-endogenous"—confirmed through such markers as abnormal sleep studies and abnormal DST.[59] (As late as 1996, Rush was demonstrating that the "endogenous/non-endogenous dichotomy" of the Research Diagnostic Criteria "was validated by the DST."[60])

In 1987, the World Health Organization Collaborative Study looked at DST results in twelve different countries from the Netherlands to Japan—this at a time when the test lay dying in the United States—concluding that "an abnormal DST response is one of the more robust biological characteristics of [major depressive] illness."[61] Almost as those lines were being penned in Geneva, Mihàly Aratò in Budapest said to Walter Brown of the DST, "I feel a kind of frustration because I strongly believe that there is something there, and I just cannot find the appropriate method to prove it."[62]

In those years catatonia was of little clinical interest and assumed to be a variety of schizophrenia. Yet a group of Hungarian researchers found in 1984 that the DST was highly positive in "catatonic schizophrenia," though unrevealing in the paranoid subtype. This was an early biological hint of schizophrenic "subtypes" so diverse as to be separate illnesses.[63]

Yet the waning interest in the DST caused such intriguing little hints to be brushed aside.

The National Institute of Mental Health held a symposium in 1983 at McMaster University in Hamilton, Ontario, on psychoneuroendocrinology. The yawning at the symposium about the DST was perceptible. Finally, Seymour Reichlin, professor of medicine at Tufts and chief of the endocrinology division of the New England Medical Center in Boston, was unable to contain his impatience.

> It has been pointed out, particularly by Dr. Carroll, that one of the most important aspects of the dexamethasone suppression test, other than the fact it is a quite reliable indicator of depression, is that it is a test of some very indirect measure of a pathological process. Nevertheless, it is a marker of an "organic" abnormality which has been confirmed in many laboratories. There are precious few of these "hard" markers in clinical psychiatry and ... it is a tremendously important thing to have something like this.[64]

A tremendously important thing, indeed. And psychiatry proceeded to lose it completely from view.

6

Trouble

"When we first started," said Walter Brown about the DST, "there were no doubters or cynics. The doubters and cynics came after there was all this brouhaha about 'Here's a diagnostic test for depression.' But in the beginning, there was a period when everybody was just tremendously excited."[1]

How did the doubters end the interest in the DST? How did a test that aroused so much excitement suddenly fall into disrepute and disappear?

In the early 1980s, partly as a consequence of *DSM-III* and of the saturation of psychopharmacology, the climate within psychiatry shifted subtly. Symptom checklists replaced an interest in psychopathology—the close observation of the patient's signs and symptoms. Barney Carroll recalled a visit to Washington University in St. Louis, where he had come from Michigan to give grand rounds:

Carroll: They brought in . . . a young black woman from East St. Louis. She had been hospitalized at that point for nine days. I talked with her, and got her version of what had led to her hospitalization. And the story briefly was: She was living in a ghetto household occupied by fifteen individuals, of whom she was the only one who had any employment. The others had some welfare money coming in, but she was the only one gainfully employed. She had several children by several different partners in the house, and she had the feeling that her life was going nowhere and that the more she struggled, the more behind she got. And she more or less used the line from that classic movie, *Network*, "I'm fed up and I'm not going to take it any more."

Interviewer: Why was she hospitalized?

Carroll: She had a screaming fit.

Interviewer: Oh, a manic episode?

Carroll: No, she wasn't manic; she was just angry. She had a screaming fit, and somebody called the police. And she screamed at the police— so the police brought her to the emergency room, and she was hospitalized. She never threatened to kill herself, she never threatened harm to anybody else, she just couldn't take it anymore.

Asked how she was feeling now, she said, "Oh, I'm great in here— there's no problem at all, I'm out of all that mess."

Interviewer: Do you think she had a psychiatric diagnosis of any kind?

Carroll: Well, this is the nub of the story. After she was taken back to the ward, we had a discussion by the group. "What is her diagnosis?" And I led off by saying, "Well, I'm very happy you brought this patient to me because I think she illustrates the difficulty of [reconciling] good clinical and criterion-based [*DSM*] diagnoses, of meshing the two. My view of this lady is that she has, if anything, an adjustment disorder, with depressed mood, of fairly short duration."

Interviewer: What did the Wash U group say?

Carroll: Well, this created great consternation at Wash U. The residents kind of were taken aback. They expected me to say, "Tick, tick, tick, tick—and this, that and the other symptom, and this adds up to a major depressive episode." And I said, "Well, nominally it may add up to a major depressive episode, just as bereavement nominally adds up to a major depressive episode—but we don't regard it as that because there are other narrative facts that weigh into the clinical decision." And they were completely unable to process that notion.[2]

A psychiatry torn adrift from concepts of narrative and context and dependent upon symptom checklists for making diagnoses would be vulnerable to the promise of a simple biological test for "depression." In addition to the symptom checklist, a positive DST assured the diagnosis. The DST spread quickly because it offered independent verification of a diagnosis, with the reassurance that a laboratory test gives the clinician.

Brown said that one reason why the DST was considered a failure was "because in the minds of some people it was too good to be true. So people wanted to poke a hole in it: it was too easy. Here's a simple test, you're going to diagnose depression, it was too good to be true."[3]

Credulousness gave way to cynicism. Clinicians attuned to the notion that psychiatry is basically list-making became vexed when a biological test, as they conceive it, reinforces this mindset and then lets them down. Perfectly understandable. But in psychiatry are we not supposed to be dealing with science and not an emotional form of checkers?

A Problem with Specificity

What evidence of imperfection surfaced? In the early 1980s, the wind started to turn against the DST as clinicians reported a lack of specificity: the "can't-rule-out" problem. In 1982 Thomas Insel and co-workers in the Clinical Neuropharmacology Branch of the NIMH administered the DST to sixteen patients with obsessive-compulsive disorder, about half of whom were also depressed. "An abnormal DST response" was recorded in six (37 percent). The authors saw this as evidence of a possible common biological substrate between obsessive-compulsive disorder and depression.[4] But the article was soon cited as evidence of the lack of specificity of the DST: the test was also positive in obsessive-compulsive disorder (overlooking that four of the six were also depressed).

Some healthy subjects had abnormal DST reactions. In 1984, a team of German psychiatrists at the Max Planck Institute for Psychiatry in Munich found that 12 percent of healthy subjects were DST non-suppressors and that the test was not able to separate endogenous depressive patients from those with other psychiatric disorders. The authors concluded, "From a clinical point of view, the DST nonsuppressors are not a homogeneous group of patients, so that the test does not contribute to a validation of clinical descriptive diagnoses." The diagnoses were made with the ICD criteria of the World Health Organization and not with *DSM*.[5]

Working with *DSM-III* definitions of major depression augured even worse for the specificity of the dexamethasone test. Most of the discouraging articles about the test relied on the *DSM* rather than the sturdier melancholia profile of the *ICD* series. One example in a sea of doubt is the report by researchers at the Veterans Administration Medical Center in Newington, Connecticut. They studied the DST in 277 inpatients "manifesting a depressive affect." Of the patients specifically with major depression, 63 percent were nonsuppressors; of other patients with a depressive affect of some kind, 32 percent were nonsuppressors. After removal of the "false positive" alcoholic and organic-brain-syndrome subjects, this gave the DST a specificity of 73 percent "for correctly diagnosing major depression in a heterogeneous group of psychiatric inpatients." The authors concluded, "The usefulness of the DST as a specific biological marker for depression appears to be poor when utilized in an inpatient setting as a differential diagnostic tool."[6]

Critics increasingly brandished these findings at Carroll. "What about your famous test now, eh?" Carroll responded that a little common sense was necessary. He had conceived the DST for melancholia, and many of these "depressive" patients were simply not melancholic. He often invoked "Bayesian logic," which meant that contextual clinical information is important for interpreting the test result. For instance, younger melancholic patients without psychotic features were unlikely to have other illnesses for which the DST was also positive, such as dementia. Named after eighteenth-century English theologian and mathematician Thomas Bayes, Bayesian logic, as applied to medical tests, means how much test results alter the probability that a patient has a given disease. In the words of two modern students, "This requires estimation of a pre-test probability that will be adjusted up or down by the test results."[7] Thus, false-positive rates did not necessarily matter, because the physician already knew that the patient probably did not have the other illnesses for which the DST may be positive. The principal use for the DST was to identify the melancholic subgroup of depressed patients rather than to distinguish melancholia from the universe of all other psychiatric diagnoses. To simplify, Carroll often used a quote of Marvin Minsky's, "When you look around a room, you expect to see tables and chairs but not a battleship."[8] Thus, the DST should not be rejected on the grounds that it was theoretically capable of identifying battleships.

Yet, in conducting a rear-guard defense, Carroll made two strategic errors. He would casually throw off a term like "Bayesian logic" to justify his position, and few psychiatrists, untrained in formal logic, knew what it meant. A standard textbook of medical statistics says, "There is another, broader definition of probability which leads to a different approach to statistics, the Bayesian school, but it is beyond the scope of this book."[9] When Carroll introduced the notion at a contentious NIMH meeting in 1982 (*see below*), it seemed "an alien construct"[10] to those present. On another occasion he scolded, "Many academic and general psychiatrists do not understand the basic theories of conditional probability or predictive value, not to mention the more advanced concepts of Bayesian theory . . . ."[11] Such a pronouncement would not have gone over well.

There was also confusion about the subject of discussion. As Walter Brown points out, when Carroll said "depression," he meant "melancholia." "He was meaning something different than what a lot of other people used it for."[12] Carroll himself was proud of the Department of Psychiatry at the University of Michigan for putting melancholia back on the radar of American psychiatry.[13] He noted in his tidy cursive script in the margin of Brown's draft of the Task Force report of September 1983: "The most powerful claim from [the Ann Arbor group] re diagnosis is use of the DST to distinguish endogenomorphic depression (or the Kraepelinian concept of melancholia) from non-endogenous depression. The implication is that the former requires somatic antidepressant treatment while the latter probably does not."[14]

The DST was in fact highly specific for melancholic depression. But a broadly defined "depression" was an imprecise concept, like "tension," "stress," or "trauma." Few clinical case presentations lack some element of dysphoria, feeling "down," sad, lacking energy, inability to experience pleasure, unhappiness, and an inability to get one's act together. These conditions were not "melancholia," and Carroll never conceived the cortisol abnormality that characterized certain biological illnesses as applying to them. Yet somehow this distinction was not clarified.

NIMH Plays a Card

The single event that tipped the scales against the DST was a workshop at the NIMH held in Bethesda, Maryland, on July 20 and 21, 1982. The genesis of this event is obscure. At that time NIMH was "flooded" with grant applications on the DST and neuroendocrine tests. It is possible that NIMH grant review officers needed guidelines. According to Carroll, the Institute felt a need to react to his 1981 article: "Oh, my God, there's all this interest swirling around out there since Carroll's publication last year, and we're NIMH, and we've got to make a policy statement!"[15] (In response to a Freedom of Information Act inquiry, NIMH informed the authors that no material relating to this workshop could be found.)

Carroll continued:

> I was ticked off because the science tradition that I developed in,
> would have said, "Keep your bloody hands off it and let the field
> sort it out." But instead we get this sort of heavy-fisted,
> interfering, pre-emptive, *consensus-building*, right—which I think
> is one of the most destructive features of current psychiatry. You
> don't see consensus-building conferences in rheumatology or
> diabetes.[16]

The conference was organized by Robert Hirschfeld, then chief of
the Center for Studies of Affective Disorders of NIMH, with Stephen
Koslow at the Neurosciences Research Branch of NIMH and David
Kupfer of the Western Psychiatric Institute in Pittsburgh. Hirschfeld
had graduated in medicine from the University of Michigan in 1968,
trained in psychiatry at Stanford, and then joined NIMH in 1972.

With the exception of Carroll and Peter Stokes at New York
Hospital, a founder of the test and author of a "historical overview" at
the workshop, there were few other clinicians who had had extensive
experience with it.[17] After the meeting, Carroll drew up a list of friends
experienced with the test who might have been invited, but were not. He
noted those who were favorably inclined "but [are] unwilling to step
forward for fear of possible repercussions." These included George
Winokur, chief of psychiatry at the University of Iowa; Paula Clayton,
chief of psychiatry at the University of Minnesota in Minneapolis; and
John Rush, of the University of Texas Southwest Medical Center at
Dallas. Carroll also listed those who were "excluded" for unclear reasons, including his friend Bob Rubin, at Harbor–UCLA Medical Center
in Torrance, California; Michael Schlesser, professor of psychiatry at
the University of Texas in Dallas; and Alan Schatzberg, then at McLean
Hospital in Belmont, Massachusetts.[18] (Schatzberg, for example, had
just come out in favor of the DST as "mov[ing] the field of psychiatry to
a more biological pole. In and of itself, this movement could prove to be
of great importance for many depressed patients who are not receiving
somatic therapies."[19])

When Carroll arrived at the workshop, he found a rather different
group of faces among those presenting papers: Donald Klein at
Columbia University, a pioneer of psychopharmacology, was invited.
Klein was involved with biological probes for panic disorder and had no
particular interest in the DST. Together with two other scholars at the

workshop, Klein reviewed the studies on specificity and found that the DST "does not seem to be a powerful differential diagnostic tool."[20]

Likewise, Peter Stokes was dubious about its specificity. Several years later, he said that "the clinical utility of the DST in psychiatry is not established."[21]

Seymour Reichlin, an endocrinologist at the New England Medical Center Hospital in Boston, thought well of the DST. Steven Targum came from across town in Washington, D.C., where he was a psychiatrist at Georgetown University School of Medicine, to tell the workshop, "The DST does not predict differential treatment response between suppressors and nonsuppressors."[22]

Fred Goodwin, scientific director of the intramural research program of NIMH, with Thomas Insel, a member of the Clinical Neuropsychopharmacology Branch at the Institute, described the importance of the normalization of test results during treatment.[23] Their report had a neutral valence, but Insel and Goodwin would shortly venture that "[t]he fundamental question about clinical application of a laboratory test is whether the test tells clinicians something that they do not already know." The DST, they concluded, alas, did not.[24]

Insel was not hostile to the DST, and his motive in writing such an unremittingly negative report is unclear. Privately, he told Alexander Glassman at the New York State Psychiatric Institute, two years later, in 1984, on the occasion of another such workshop of the APA, "The story reads now as follows: of 143 DST nonsuppressors, 36 failed to normalize, and of this cohort of 36, 32 relapsed within 1–6 months. By contrast, of the 107 who converted to a normal DST, only 10 relapsed during the same intervals.... The evidence as it stands, certainly suggests that a positive (not a negative) DST has some prognostic value."[25] This was a vote of confidence for the DST as a predictor of relapse. These data were unfortunately never made public.

Finally, James Maas of the University of Texas at San Antonio spoke of other possible biological markers in depression, and Herb Meltzer at the Illinois State Psychiatric Institute in Chicago talked about "technical issues," dwelling upon "factors causing false positive DST."[26]

A number of other scholars discussed these papers. But nowhere, either in the brief summaries of the discussion or in the published papers, was any glint of enthusiasm for the DST discerned. The contributions ranged from the sharply negative to the indifferent claim that the DST might be worth investigating scientifically, along with other neuroendocrine tests (a valid claim), but that clinically using the test was a waste of time.

Carroll gave "an overview of the clinical utility of the DST," and was allocated forty-five minutes, much longer than any other presenter. But, evidently feeling his back against the wall, he permitted an irascible side of his disposition to emerge. "It was really Barney against everybody," said Walter Brown, present as a discussant.[27]

Bob Spitzer, also a discussant, clashed with Carroll. Carroll later said that he had offered data to support his views, but "Spitzer was in the room, and he said, 'We're not going to deal with this!'"

Then Carroll "challenged Spitzer." "I said, 'Well, in effect what I'm offering is external validation of the classic melancholia construct, and if you don't want to buy that, Bob, then why don't you give us an external validation of your construct?' And at that point [Spitzer] said, 'No, it's too early to do that, but we're going to deal with my construct, because that's the way I've decided."[28]

Carroll said that Insel "was adamant that because he had found positive tests in OCD [obsessive compulsive disorder], this [test] couldn't possibly be any use in depression." Carroll claimed that Insel was highly vocal in his views and swayed a number of participants: "He jumped up and down on a soap box about it."[29]

Carroll left the workshop in a fury and was, he said, not asked to contribute to the conference volume. Walter Brown later said, "During this period Barney was difficult to deal with. I mean, people didn't want to piss him off, but the discussions were not carried out in an atmosphere of affective neutrality. (*Laughter*) And he was prickly."[30]

The workshop could hardly have augured worse for the DST. Few would have seen the reports of the proceedings brought out by NIMH.[31] The summary that Hirschfeld published in the *Journal of the American Medical Association* on October 28, 1983, however, received wide circulation. Even useful aspects of the DST mentioned at the workshop were hedged into disfavor. Hirschfeld trivialized Insel's favorable assessment of the DST in predicting relapse and simply said the whole question "needs further study."[32] "The DST is a useful research tool, but at this time there are no clear indications for its *routine* use in the diagnosis or clinical management of depression." If there are no indications for its routine use, then there are no indications for its use. The DST was deemed not useful and could be disregarded.

These were difficult days for Carroll as he watched the gathering storm. At the December 1982 meeting of the American College of

Neuropsychopharmacology (ACNP) in San Juan, Tom Detre, director of the Western Psychiatric Institute in Pittsburgh, had arranged a symposium on the DST. John Rush, then associate professor at Southwestern Medical School in Dallas, though not yet an ACNP member, attended and gave a paper. Carroll did not attend, and in January of 1983, Rush reported to Carroll on how things had gone. It was not a report Carroll would have found thrilling. "It was only modestly attended because it was a 9:00 P.M. evening program." Herb Meltzer, then director of the Laboratory of Biological Psychiatry at the Illinois State Psychiatric Institute in Chicago, turned up at the symposium and was querulous: "Herb Meltzer had significant questions about the specificity of the test [as Rush had used it]." Rush tried to cool him down by explaining that in patients with minor infections and the like, false positives could occur. "Herb seemed to be partly satisfied with that idea."[33] But not really. This was another bad sign.

"Bright and Shiny Toy"?

In the meantime, the APA was wrestling with biological psychiatry. In 1979, in the throes of debate over the forthcoming third edition of the *DSM*, the Association's board of directors recommended the creation of an Office of Research. Until the actual opening of such an office, research issues at APA would be the responsibility of an unnamed staffer, who, late in 1982 or early in 1983, appears to have asked Alexander ("Sandy") Glassman at Columbia University to chair a task force on laboratory tests in psychiatry.[34] Though the remit was apparently broad, it was the DST that this task force was supposed to analyze.

Even from the composition of the task force it was clear there was trouble ahead. Among the members were Barney Carroll, whose appointment Harold Pincus (who took over the Office of Research in 1985) later characterized as a "mistake." "He was," said Pincus in an interview, "so personally identified that he couldn't be objective."[35]

Also on the task force were Ross Baldessarini and George Arana of McLean Hospital, who, during the deliberations of the task force, kept up a steady stream of articles hostile to the DST and were probably among the country's most articulate and determined opponents of the procedure. Baldessarini had never done the DST, but Arana, a fellow at the Mailman Laboratories of McLean Hospital between 1979 and 1983, did routinely conduct it. In May of 1983, in an article in the *Archives of General Psychiatry*, they put the idea of biomedical "tests" in psychiatry in ironical quotation marks. They claimed, "The DST and other endocrinological tests being developed for use in evaluating depression are limited in sensitivity, and their specificity, when applied to acutely, severely ill psychiatric patients, is not secure."[36] Putting Carroll and Baldessarini and his students together on a task force designed to evaluate Carroll's test was a recipe for disaster.

Other members played less rancorous roles. There was Walter Brown, of whom Arana recalls, "Walter was even-handed about it. He wasn't grinding an axe." Also on the task force were John Davis of the Illinois State Psychiatric Institute, David Greenblatt of Tufts University, Gerald Klerman at the Payne-Whitney Clinic at Cornell University (who was virtually invisible during the proceedings), Paul Orsulak of the University of Texas Southwestern Medical Center, Joe Schildkraut of Harvard (originator of the "norepinephrine theory of depression" in 1965), and Richard Shader, also of Harvard. Consultants such as Alan Schatzberg and Martin Teicher came and went.

As the task force began its meetings, the battle lines, Arana recalled in an interview with one of the authors, were quite clear.

Arana: Barney was clearly strongly wanting us to publish a positive paper, that we have a marker here. Alan Schatzberg at that point was enchanted with the test also, and he was running a depression research unit at McLean, so he was seeing a lot more integrity of the test in that setting.

Fink: And Ross?

Arana: Ross was saying, "I have doubts about this test right now, because I don't see what it contributes to differential [diagnosis]. And I don't want to tout this as the first of the great biological tests in psychiatry, because we've done this kind of thing for the last fifty years and fallen on our faces over and over again." He was talking about being cautious . . . . I don't know if you know Ross?

Fink: Yes, I know Ross.

Arana: He's a very critical person.[37]

The task force worked speedily. By October of 1983, Walter Brown had drafted an initial report, which Carroll, by now having moved from Michigan to Duke, found "inadequate in its scope, misleading in its conceptualization of the nosological issues, and condescending in its tone." Carroll also charged that Brown had quoted selectively from the negative reports in the literature.[38] But there was another way to still Carroll's objections: ask Baldessarini and Arana to write the report. By June of 1984 they had commenced work,[39] and in September they offered a draft to the task force. In the meantime, as we saw in the previous chapter, in December of 1984 Arana and Baldessarini let fly another blast against the DST in the *American Journal of Psychiatry*, suggesting that DST results were due to differences in metabolizing dexamethasone rather than to true differences in cortisol on the HPA axis:[40] that the results of the test were artifacts, in other words.

Carroll fired back with an article in the *Journal of Clinical Psychiatry* in 1985, slamming his critics as "credulous" and "confused."[41]

The stage was now set for a donnybrook within the badly divided committee. This took place in May of 1985 at the annual meeting of the APA in Dallas. Glassman presented a draft document to the task force, based largely on Baldessarini and Arana's views, as rounded out by Shader and Glassman. Shortly after the Dallas meeting, Glassman wrote to Brown, "Unfortunately, there was some significant disagreement about whether this document, in its outline form, was satisfactory." There were two camps: "Arana, Shader, and Glassman felt that they could live with this document . . . . [The DST] represented a very weak test with respect to diagnostic specificity and there was concern that its implications for treatment could easily be misinterpreted." On the other hand, "Carroll, Shildkraut [*sic*] and Orsulak took the position that this report would be read as a glass 'half empty' rather than a glass 'half full.' They felt that it was important to psychiatry in general that the report be much more positive in its tone." It was decided that Carroll and Schildkraut would prepare an alternative version; the task force would meet in Boston in September to reconcile the two versions.[42]

At the Boston meeting, the task force agreed that Glassman himself should reconcile the competing versions. Brown wrote Glassman afterwards, "[I] could find no blood on the floor, so I think you are to be congratulated."[43] Glassman reported later in September of 1985 to the APA's Council on Research, "The Task Force has been struggling with a report . . . for the past year." Glassman's own version would be circulated in hopes of an agreement. Herbert Pardes, chair of the Council, added pointedly that "if the Task Force can't agree on a statement their report should perhaps reflect that fact."[44] APA's impatience with the squabbling task force was palpable.

But tensions on the task force grew worse, not better. The definitive attack on the DST by Baldessarini and Arana, evidently based on their own draft for the task force, was published in the *Archives of General Psychiatry* in December 1985. The basic argument turned on the inadequacy of the DST for learning anything of importance about "major depression." The best that could be concluded of the DST, they said, was that it "encourages the search for other simple biological measures."[45]

Carroll was maddened by the piece. He told Glassman several days after it appeared, referring to similar tables of specificity data that Baldessarini and Arana had prepared for the task force:

> I'm sorry to have to say that there are *MAJOR* problems with the numbers that George and Ross have come up with in their summary tables.... As I recall, they seemed all gung ho to do this job [prepare the tables for the task force], and indeed volunteered. Otherwise, I would have done it myself. But, because of the general tendency of the Task Force members to see me as biased, I let them go ahead. Having now seen the result, I must say in all candor that they did a lousy job.[46]

On the following day, December 30, Carroll sent Glassman a detailed critique of the Baldessarini-Arana draft report for the Task Force. They had relied too much upon *DSM-III* diagnoses, said Carroll. "I am disturbed by the lack of scientific thoughtfulness in the review as a whole. To do justice to our collective IQs, we should avoid taking the hook, line and sinker position that DSM III is an acceptable 'gold standard' by which the DST can be evaluated." Carroll considered the Baldessarini-Arana effort largely valueless.[47] (He also sent a detailed critique of the *Archives* article to the editors, which they did not publish.)

Almost three years had now passed since the task force took up its work. In April of 1986, Glassman penned a third version of the report and circulated it for comment. Sounding sick to death of the whole business, he said he would submit the report to the task force for a vote! Glassman then forwarded what he had written to the APA Reference Committee as the final report.

"Dear Sandy, I am mad as hell with you because you didn't do what you said you were going to do," Carroll responded on June 12, 1986. "You assured me in Washington last month that you would send me promptly the final text of the task force report. You haven't done that." Carroll threatened to damn the report publicly and told

Glassman he was forwarding a copy of his letter to Herbert Pardes, chair of the Council on Research, and Harold Pincus, the new head of the APA Office of Research.[48]

There was more to-ing and fro-ing. Pincus called Carroll, trying to get him to stay on board. Finally, at the end of June, 1986, Glassman threw his hands in the air. "I think we should send the report forward with or without Barney's approval," he told the task force.[49]

Three weeks later, Carroll told Glassman he found Glassman's letter to the task force "insulting to me, distorted and self-serving." Carroll said he found the quality of the report that Glassman had forwarded to APA "disgraceful." "It contains still a number of stupidities, misleading statements, amateurish passages and omissions. And the references!" Carroll said, "If you go ahead with the report as is, then I insist that you remove my name from it."[50]

Harold Pincus had now completely lost patience with Carroll. At a meeting of the Council on September 10, 1986, after being briefed on the ill-fated task force's wrangling, he said words to the effect, "Carroll can accept, not accept, drop from process." He asked Herb Pardes to lay down an ultimatum.[51]

There was much more discussion, and the final report was not submitted to the Board of Trustees of the APA until December of 1986. It turned out to be an anticlimax, because the report was never published in full. Instead, a summary appeared in the *American Journal of Psychiatry* in October 1987, offering a discouraging opinion of the DST: "Due to the limited sensitivity of the DST, . . . the usefulness of the test is not high when a patient is either very likely or very unlikely to have a major affective disorder." Given the probability of such a disorder, "a positive DST result is reassuring."[52] For believers in the utility of the DST, this conclusion was dismaying: Few clinicians would have felt it necessary to ask their patients to pay several hundred extra dollars for "reassurance" of a diagnosis they already believed clinically to be correct.

To be sure, the report said the test might predict worsening in patients who had apparently recovered. But apart from that, "The task force found no incontrovertible role for the DST in current clinical practice."[53]

That was the end. Carroll had done his best to defend the test he had introduced to psychiatry, but was swamped with studies showing that it had low specificity in "major depression," a disease that was so ill-defined as to offer no guide to prognosis or treatment.

In the postmortem, Baldessarini was scornful of all the "biological tests." He said of the task force in an interview, "There was a lot of discussion in that panel, sometimes rather heated. Some members were betting the ranch that biological testing was going to revolutionize the industry, and were very invested and enthusiastic. They didn't want to hear critical comments. It was one of the first times in my career of being amazed at how personal scientific undertakings can become."[54] Baldessarini was right to the extent that the task force held at least one meeting without inviting Carroll, as Walter Brown said, "to allow 'freer discussion' or something like that."[55]

Twenty years later, Carroll was still bitter.

Interviewer: So the deck was just totally stacked?

Carroll: There you have it. (*Laughter*) Pardes called and threatened me, that if I didn't put my name on it, things would be even worse for me.... He said, "My advice is, stay on board with the rest of the group."

Interviewer: Which you did?

Carroll: I finally allowed that to happen, yeah.

What did the task force do wrong? we asked Carroll. He did not respond that their major blunder was not listening to him. Instead, he brought up Walter Brown's 1985 finding of lack of placebo response in DST nonsuppressors: The members of the task force should have asked why drug versus placebo differences were so great with DST nonsuppressors. Baldessarini and Arana, he said, had fixated on the wrong point, which was why the DST failed to predict treatment response and to assure diagnosis.

Carroll declared, "If you ask the question the right way, and say 'What is the drug/placebo difference in response rate'? then the scales fall away. For DST positives, the drug response rate is 70 percent; the placebo response rate is about 10 percent. For the DST negatives, the drug response rate is about 60 percent, and the placebo response rate is about 50 percent. You get it?"[56]

Somehow, this scientifically interesting question was never asked in the rumpus surrounding the task force, just as this question also was never asked: "What is going on with these depressed patients who have in common high-serum cortisol as a biological abnormality?" John Greden, chair of psychiatry at Michigan, said in an interview in 2003, "Our country got a little too occupied with the idea that the dexamethasone suppression test might be a lab test. In actuality...it was really a reflection of what was going on in the brain."[57] In a dismaying reprise of the *DSM-III* process, the entire APA task force on biological tests offers an example of how committee-drawn classifications based on consensus can trump science. Carroll, the only member of the committee not in tune with its consensus politics, turned out to be right in the end.

Did the task force sound the death-knell of the DST or merely write the epitaph of a procedure that was already dead? Baldessarini said later, "My recollection was that George Arana and I found a dead body by the roadside and merely wrote an epitaph for the gravestone."[58] Walter Brown agreed with this assessment. He saw the task force report published in the *American Journal of Psychiatry* in 1987 as urging the psychiatric community to suspend judgment until all the information was in. "But it was too late. The tide had turned."[59]

Decline

The DST flooded out of psychiatry as quickly as it had flooded in. "Today," said Walter Brown in 1990, "it would be difficult to find any psychiatric setting where the DST is used, other than as a test for Cushing's syndrome."[60]

Bob Rubin recalls how the DST ended at the Harbor–UCLA Medical Center in Torrance, California, where he was a staff psychiatrist in the 1970s and 1980s: "It was a tough test to do. You needed site nurses to do blood sampling. There was the question of the form of dex. We always used the elixir. Our residents lost interest when they went out into practice. The new cohort of residents heard bad-mouthing of it by the senior clinicians. Inertia set in, then they gave up on it."[61] So at Harbor–UCLA it was not a sudden, dramatic decision prompted by any specific journal article, but rather like the air leaking out of a tire.

Ross Baldessarini was not upset at the decline of the procedure and scorned his colleagues for their vulnerability to what he considered fads. "I think it's like a lot of other things in biological psychiatry. There have been waves of enthusiasm, and when an idea or a technology is relatively new, it's a bright and shiny toy, and people play with it for a few years, and then find the limitations and they get bored. By then there's a new game in town, and they move on."[62]

Psychiatry turned from the DST, revulsed. By the mid-1980s, the group of investigators in Budapest who had been keen on the test was having a hard time getting their research published. In 1986, Mihály Arató wrote to Walter Brown, "I think that everybody is fed up with DST so for a while it is hard to publish anything."[63]

In the decline of the DST, the little adventitious moments that make history intermingled with the grand currents. Barney Carroll's personality played a role, but so did big changes in the medical and political landscape. Medicine in the 1980s was in transition.

"The *Zeitgeist* changed," said Carroll in 2005. "Reimbursement is difficult now. Between then and now something else happened, called managed care. And reimbursement for the $250 test is not as simple as it used to be in the '80s." He added, "I think when it really died was when the world realized that you should have dexamethasone levels [in the late 1980s, as well as cortisol levels]. And then that intersected with managed care, and then when the potential cost of doing the test got to be over a certain psychological threshold, then people said, 'The payoff isn't worth what it's going to cost.'"[64]

But did it die in the world of science, in academic psychiatry?

"The whole neuroendocrine strategy failed," said Charlie Nemeroff, chair of psychiatry at Emory University in Atlanta. "If we can understand how neuroendocrine secretion is altered in illness, we can infer brain changes."[65] But this promise was never realized.

Carroll added, "NIMH has steered away from neuroendocrine studies in general, in favor of translational research, and that was especially true under Steven Hyman [1996–2002]. So that to get a pure neuroendocrine grant funded through the '90s was quite difficult." Uriel Halbreich, a former collaborator of Edward Sachar's at Columbia and now at the New York State University at Buffalo, confirmed this in an interview: "People say, 'Well, nobody wants to fund that anymore so I guess I'll move on.'"[66]

Did any influential figures continue to advocate the DST?

Carroll said, "I think the bottom line is: No champion stood up for it, besides me. And I didn't want to develop into another Joe Schildkraut, who was flogging a dead horse [the norepinephrine theory of depression]."[67]

In 1997, Carroll wrote to Don Klein, "Very good to hear from you and to learn about your latest undertaking with the new journal *Treatment*. I appreciate the invitation to write an article on the DST but I am going to turn you down because I have decided that anything I write will be discounted."[68]

And so the last public advocate of the DST fell silent.

Postscript, by Max Fink

Neither I nor Michael Alan Taylor was well acquainted with this history when we undertook *Melancholia*.[69] We were not included in the NIMH or APA assessments, nor were we committed to the DST or against it. Like other academic researchers and teachers, we moved on to other interests. I continued to use the DST to teach residents about the biology of depression, the mechanism of ECT, and for some consultations where the question of ECT was the focus, to offer the DST as a "test of prognosis and remission."

In reviewing the literature for *Melancholia*, including the writings of Carroll, Baldessarini and Arana, Brown and others, we became increasingly impressed with the validity of the Carroll conclusion—that the DST was a measure of a cerebral abnormality, and cortisol abnormality was central to "melancholia."

I was requesting the DST in selected inpatients, and in 1996 the department chair, Fritz Henn, called me and asked whether I could fund the DST from my research funds. Insurers were refusing to reimburse the cost of the test, based on the APA position. From then on, the test was done mainly in our research cases.

But when we reviewed the DST literature from 2003 through 2005, we were impressed with the number of studies that found the DST positive in severely depressed, melancholic patients. The reversion to normal was predictive of a good outcome. Failure to normalize predicted relapse and, more compellingly, was a harbinger of suicide. We saw that the test was discarded because it was matched against an unreliable and unstable diagnosis of "major depression" and because of the fallacious splitting of a single manic-depressive illness into "major depression" and "bipolar disorder." We were sufficiently convinced that the DST reflected a biological abnormality of clinical significance that we urged its use to define melancholia, as a measure of remission and relapse, and of suicide risk.

We recognized that the test was imperfect and needed "work." The DEX-CRF modification (see Chapter 7), serum levels of dexamethasone, and other variations warranted study. But as it stands, the DST is better than its popular reputation. Its discard was an inexcusable error.

7

"The Most Exciting Development in the Endocrine Study of Depression"

The figures who have appeared up to now have mainly been psychiatrists. But the study of neuroendocrinology began in departments of anatomy and zoology, far from the clinical beds of the psychiatric wards. It is the discipline focused on the relationship between the hypothalamus and the rest of the body, rather than, as in endocrine psychiatry, the relationship of mental illness and the thyroid and adrenal axes. Neuroendocrinology ended up dominated by endocrinologists, most interested in the reproductive hormones rather than the glucocorticoids of the adrenal cortex. Yet the efforts of neuroendocrinology have produced therapeutic benefits for the psychiatric clinic.

The Rise of Neuroendocrinology

In the beginning, the crucial question was: Did the hypothalamus control the pituitary? And if so, how?

In 1928, Ernst Scharrer, a graduate student in the department of zoology of the University of Munich, discovered, in the words of his wife and fellow scientist Berta Scharrer, that "certain hypothalamic neurons specialize in secretory activity to a degree comparable to that of endocrine gland cells."[1] By 1940, Ernst and Berta Scharrer were safely ensconced at the Rockefeller Institute for Medical Research in New York, away from persecution in Germany; their 1940 article on secretory cells within the hypothalamus fortified the doctrine of neurosecretion[2]—that hormones provided the link between the central nervous system and the endocrine system. As Chandler Brooks, professor of physiology at New York's Downstate Medical Center in the 1960s, later observed, "This started the work which became a major contribution to the founding of neuroendocrinology: the demonstration that ADH [antidiuretic hormone] and oxytocin are produced by neurons."[3]

But what was the chemistry of this traffic in messages? In 1931, Ulf von Euler and John Gaddum, at the National Institute for Medical Research in the London suburb of Hampstead, discovered the first peptide hormone in horse small intestine. They called it "preparation P."[4] (They were unable to characterize it chemically.) Only decades later were peptide hormones discovered in the central nervous system, and that was accomplished with the technology of radioimmunoassay (RIA), a technology that von Euler and Gaddum did not possess. This was the beginning of the "peptide era" in neuroscience: the hormones of brain and pituitary were peptides, low-molecular-weight compounds composed of amino acids.

Endocrine communication is governed by the principle of negative feedback: An increase in the amount of a circulating hormone, such as cortisol or thyroxine, alerts the anterior pituitary and hypothalamus that too much is being manufactured and that it is time to turn off the flow. In the winter of 1930, Dorothy Price, a research assistant in the department of zoology of the University of Chicago, became intrigued by the problem of "sex hormone antagonism." As she later asked rhetorically, "What controlled the secretion of anterior pituitary hormones and shielded the gonads from overstimulation?" She tried to make sense of the data produced by her laboratory chief, zoologist Carl Moore: "After dinner that night, I sat down at my desk and thought! I simplified the problem by reducing the results to essentially three statements . . . . Then, quite suddenly a plausible explanation occurred to me. The secretion of male hormone depended upon gonadotropic hormone from the pituitary . . . ." She worked out the logic of a self-regulating system. "I did not call this brainchild of mine a theory or a hypophysis [sic—she meant hypothesis] and I certainly did not anticipate that it would come to be known as a negative feedback system. I thought it a beautiful and logical scheme ...."[5] Later in 1930, she and Moore published the finding, the first untangling of endocrine interactions.[6]

Palms for pinning down the chemical nature of the communication between hypothalamus and pituitary belong to Wolfgang Bargmann and Geoffrey Harris. In 1949, Bargmann, professor of anatomy in the war-ravaged University of Kiel, examined slides from a dog brain stained with a chromalum-hematoxylin-phloxin technique that his colleague at Kiel, endocrinologist Werner Creutzfeldt, had just introduced for diabetes: "When I took the first look through the microscope—the slides still being wet—I was lucky enough to perceive at once a selectively stained neuronal system, extending uninterruptedly from the nuclei supraopticus and paraventricularis [in the hypothalamus] to the neural lobe of the hypophysis [posterior lobe of the pituitary]."[7] Bargmann published the finding immediately in a journal that he edited; as he observed, this obviated the need to deal with any objections from an anti-neurosecretionist editorial board.[8] This was the first research to demonstrate the endocrine nature of the hypothalamic connection to the posterior pituitary.

It was, however, the more sustained and influential work of Geoffrey Harris, professor of physiology first at Cambridge and then at the Maudsley Hospital in London, that definitively established that the secretions of the hypothalamus controlled the anterior pituitary gland; the pituitary was not a master gland acting of its own accord but rather the head butler in a mansion controlled by the brain. Born in 1913, Harris had been a brilliant student at Cambridge in the natural sciences. He qualified in medicine in 1939, becoming a demonstrator in anatomy at Cambridge. Chandler Brooks, who met Harris in 1938 in Zurich during the International Physiological Congress, recalls him as "a very friendly, strong, determined young man." Brooks's own knowledge of the portal system connecting hypothalamus and anterior pituitary was soon outstripped by that of Harris.[9]

In 1947, intent upon demonstrating the anatomical connections between hypothalamus and anterior pituitary, Harris examined the venous drainage of the median eminence of the hypothalamus.[10] Realizing that physiological techniques were now called for, in 1948 he moved to the physiology department at Cambridge and electrically stimulated the hypothalamus to observe its downstream effects. Studying the initiation of ovulation in rabbits, he established that the anterior pituitary (unlike the posterior pituitary) did not respond to the tiny electrical probes he installed, but the hypothalamus did. Geoff Raisman,

who has studied Harris's work closely, concludes, "This led to the important conclusion that the ovulatory signal generated by stimulating the
central nervous system (CNS) must have passed from the hypothalamus to
the pituitary."[11] But how?

Indeed, the link turned out to be vascular rather than nervous. In a
key contribution with Cambridge anatomist John Davis Green in 1949,
Harris demonstrated that blood moved from the median eminence to
the pituitary.[12] In 1950, working with Dora Jacobsohn of Lund University in Sweden, he established that a rich vascular network, capable of
regeneration, linked the hypothalamus to the anterior pituitary.[13] The
portal system is a circulatory network connecting capillary bed to
capillary bed going from the hypothalamus down to the pituitary that
had not been known before.

Jacobsohn went back to Lund, and in 1951, Harris and Jacobsohn,
their two laboratories collaborating, showed in hypophysectomized
adult rats that "grafts of anterior pituitary tissue placed under the
median eminence but not elsewhere, may prevent any marked atrophy
of the adrenal glands." This constituted, the authors said, "good evidence in support of the view that the secretion of the adrenocorticotrophic hormone [ACTH] is under hypothalamic control."[14] (Harris
had already given similar evidence in 1950 in research with Jacob
("Jack") de Groot on "hypothalamic control of the anterior pituitary
gland and blood lymphocytes."[15])

Harris often realized these advances in collaboration with the
young researchers now flocking to his laboratory. Seymour Reichlin,
a neuroendocrinologist at Tufts University in Medford, Massachusetts,
recalled of Harris, "He reserved for himself the most challenging
technical problems, such as section of the pituitary stalk or placement
of electrodes, and the more difficult the problem the more he enjoyed
it." As for committee work, always a plague in academia, Harris
shunned it. Said Reichlin, "He once counseled me to never do a
good job on a committee, otherwise I would be asked to devote more
time to administrative chores. He followed his own counsel well in
these matters."[16]

In 1952, Harris accepted the chair of physiology in the University
of London at the Maudsley Hospital. The department was housed
in "huts" on the hospital grounds. Despite rather primitive working
conditions, Harris's laboratory attracted students from all over the
world, for neuroendocrinology was exploding as an academic discipline.
The capstone of this phase of Harris's career was his 1955 book *Neural*

Control of the Pituitary Gland, bringing together evidence from a wide range of experiments. The book concluded, "There can be little doubt that vascularization of anterior pituitary tissue by the hypophysial portal system is necessary for the maintenance and control of normal activity of this gland."[17]

The center of gravity of research in neuroendocrinology then passed from the Old World to the New. Montreal became a lively *entrepôt* of neuroendocrine work. Arthur Mirsky, who later tried to combine psychoanalysis and endocrinology at Cincinnati and Pittsburgh, graduated from McGill in 1931. Selye was in Montreal. After the Second World War, the psychoendocrine scene in Montreal turned about Murray Saffran, a 1949 McGill biochemistry graduate who lectured in psychiatry at the Allan Memorial Institute.

In 1955 Saffran and his student Andrew Schally, a Polish-born scientist educated at McGill, reported evidence that "release of a factor" in the hypothalamus was responsible for the pituitary gland's secretion of ACTH.[18] They called it CRF.[19] In the same year Roger Guillemin and Barry Rosenberg at Baylor University College of Medicine in Houston reported a similar finding. Guillemin, a French physician who had earned a Ph.D. in physiology from the University of Montreal in 1952—rubbing elbows with fellow student Saffran— "postulated that there exists some hypothalamic-hypophysiotropic mediator involved in ACTH release."[20] (Interestingly, despite the indissoluble bond that exists between the names of Selye and Montreal, Guillemin developed his approach to research in opposition to Selye.[21]) For Guillemin and Schally, this was the beginning of the trail that led to the summit of neuroendocrinology, the discovery of the hypothalamic releasing factors. Between 1955 and 1968, nine other hypothalamic releasing factors were uncovered.[22]

Yet a neuroendocrinological race to the summit turned out to be a much more American than Canadian story. Basic research in neuroendocrinology in the United States, as well as in many other medical specialties, surged to world-class standing in the years after the Second World War. The United States surpassed German-speaking Europe as the world's medical epicenter, powered by the enormous amounts of money that the NIH were now pumping into basic science and enriched with the migration of Jewish scientists from lands scorched by the Holocaust to the safety of North America (Scharrer became, for example, professor of anatomy at Albert Einstein College of Medicine in New York; Dora Jacobsohn, to be sure, landed in Sweden, not the

United States, but the point of finding safety and contributing to endocrine science is made.)

On the neuroendocrine side, essential was the discovery of an assay
for spotting these peptide releasing factors, measured in the blood in
parts per million. In the mid-1950s at the Bronx Veterans Hospital,
physicist Rosalyn Yalow, in charge of the radioisotope service, and
internist Solomon Berson were doing research with psychiatric patients
who had had insulin coma therapy.[23]

> We soon deduced from the retarded rate of disappearance of
> insulin from the circulation of insulin-treated subjects that all
> these patients develop antibodies to the animal insulins. In
> studying the reaction of insulin with antibodies, we appreciated
> that we had developed a tool with the potential for measuring
> circulating insulin. It took several more years of work to transform
> the concept into the reality of its practical application to the
> measurement of plasma insulin in man.

Said Yalow: "The era of radioimmunoassay (RIA) can be said to
have begun in 1959."[24]

The spread of RIA to psychiatry was swift. In the summer of
1960, Edward Sachar, then a research fellow at Walter Reed
Hospital, wrote to his brother David, "It became clear at the
scientific congress I attended in Europe that our Walter Reed
group is so fantastically far out ahead of any other work in this
area in the world that other investigators simply shake their heads
when I showed the slides. . . . This month our chemists put the
finishing touches on a superbly sensitive immunochemical method
for measuring blood insulin; growth hormone should be ready by
the winter."[25]

Several years later, psychiatrist Walter Brown served a two-year
fellowship in neuroendocrinology under the auspices of the Foundations
Fund for Research in Psychiatry, consisting of a basic-science year at
Yale and a clinical year at Mount Sinai in New York. He recalled RIA as
"making it possible to measure very minute levels of hormones fairly
simply. Before that, there were all these kinds of bioassays—if you
wanted to know how much prolactin somebody had, you injected a
mouse and measured their mammary glands or ovaries—and there
were only sort of biological measures of hormones. But now you could
actually measure the level in the blood."[26] Robert Rubin reminds us that

at the very beginning of RIA the assays were not as specific as they later became:

> Non-biologically active fragments, especially of polypeptide hormones, and other closely related molecules that had different biological activity, such as steroid hormones, were recognized by the antibody, in addition to the primary hormone.... Today, most chemical assays are quite specific, e.g. the RIA for cortisol measures that steroid only, and the ACTH 1–39 immunoradiometric assay measures the biologically active intact molecule and not inactive pieces that also are recognized by the ACTH RIA.[27]

It was not RIA but other sophisticated biochemical techniques that permitted Guillemin and Schally in the fall of 1969, working in separate centers, to isolate and identify the chemical structure of TRH (also called TRF for "factor" rather than "hormone"), a kind of master hormone produced in many parts of the brain that keeps body and brain alike in equilibrium. Schally's laboratory at Tulane School of Medicine in New Orleans "isolated 2.8 mg of TRH from 100,000 pig hypothalami."[28] Guillemin's lab at Baylor College of Medicine in Houston purified TRH from "300,000 sheep hypothalamus fragments." Guillemin later said that, "The isolation and characterization of TRF [TRH] was ... the turning point which separated doubt—and often confusion, from unquestionable knowledge. It was of such heuristic significance that I can say that neuroendocrinology became an established science on that event."[29] Guillemin, Schally, and Yalow shared a Nobel Prize in 1977. Berson had sadly passed on. (There is a story, possibly apocryphal, that at the Nobel ceremony Schally's citation was handed to Guillemin and vice versa, leading Guillemin to comment, "Ah, so confusion [about the first discoverer] reigns to the end.")

Once the structure of TRH was known, it was easily synthesized. Radiotagged TRH opened the door to the interior of the hypothalamus. The same held true for the other hypothalamic releasing factors as they steadily became identified. It was now possible to trace the relationship among the brain, the pituitary, and the hormones of the endocrine system. Art Prange, professor of psychiatry at the UNC who pioneered the thyroid dimension of endocrine psychiatry, said in 1998, "The significance of the discovery of TRH went far beyond the description of yet another hormone. It was the first to be identified of the elusive hormonal connections between the brain and the anterior pituitary gland, which could no longer be regarded as the master gland.... Neuroendocrinology, rooted in animal research, gained a new and expanded definition; it became the premier science basic to psychoendocrinology."[30]

Psychoendocrinology Takes Off

These discoveries in the basic sciences quickened psychiatric interest in the endocrine system. "Psychoendocrine" meant peptides. What had been classical endocrine psychiatry acquired a different aspect once the brain rather than the pituitary gland became the prime mover. In 1967, Dorothy Krieger and Howard Krieger, at the Mount Sinai School of Medicine in New York, offered experimental evidence that a circadian rise in corticosteroid secretion could be suppressed by atropine, an anticholinergic agent; this suggested that "cholinergic mechanisms are involved in the release of ACTH."[31] Interest was building in neurotransmitters, and this was evidence that the endocrine system and the neurotransmitter steering of the brain were directly linked.

Here is the big picture: In the 1970s, psychiatry was leaving psychoanalysis behind and turning to brain biology as the cause of the major psychiatric diseases. In the search for brain markers, we have already reviewed interest in the DST. Yet this hunger for markers went much deeper. In 1970, Eli Robins and Sam Guze of Washington University in St. Louis, one of the piston schools of biological psychiatry, said that "[a] fully validated diagnostic classification will probably also require laboratory studies."[32] This became a banner under which the search for psychoendocrine markers went forward.

The problem was that previous research, done with relatively primitive measurements of circulating glucocorticoids, had produced puzzling and contradictory results. As David McClure and Robert Cleghorn, psychiatrists at McGill University, pointed out in 1968, "An apparent paradox has ... arisen with regard to the endocrine findings in depressive illness. Some investigators postulate a state of hyperadrenocorticism while others postulate a state of relative adrenocortical hypofunction in severe depression."[33] Which was it? Could the newly discovered releasing factors cast light?

Research got going. At NIMH, Martin Katz was chief of extramural clinical research (vetting grants to academic applicants as opposed to intramural NIMH staff scientists). At a conference on "the psychobiology of the depressive illnesses" that he organized in 1969 at Williamsburg, Virginia, David Hamburg offered conclusions on future directions of research. "Since we are concerned with the brain and behavior," he said, "we want to know whether hormones and their metabolites enter brain and affect behavior."[34] In the decade to come, the psychoendocrine answer would be "Yes!"

The standard procedure was to challenge the endocrine system, then follow the reverberations about the brain and body with RIA measures. Given the primitive state of research on the hypothalamic releasing factors in the early 1970s, investigators looked at pituitary peptide hormones such as growth hormone, inferring from them what the hypothalamus might be doing. In 1971, Edward Sachar and his colleagues at Montefiore Hospital injected insulin into 13 severely depressed patients and measured the growth-hormone (GH) response with RIA. In five patients, the GH response to hypoglycemia was "deficient"—later investigators preferred the term "blunted"—a deficiency that lessened with recovery.[35] Evidently, the hypothalamic response to hypoglycemia was blocked in hospitalized depressed patients.

A burst of research along these lines strengthened the conviction that neurotransmitters affected secretion along the HPA axis. In 1974, in an editorial in *Psychological Medicine,* James Gibbons at the University of Newcastle on Tyne summarized the findings. Norepinephrine and serotonin inhibited the hypothalamic secretion of CRH (and thus of ACTH and cortisol); dopaminergic neurons inhibited the secretion of prolactin; and norephinephrine-secreting neurons blunted the secretion of growth hormone. Gibbons wrote, "This type of investigation, combining neuropharmacological and endocrine techniques, may enable us to tease out disturbed hypothalamic functions in man. This prospect is the most exciting development in the endocrine study of depression."[36] In severe depression, the normal endocrine responses of the brain were dysregulated.

What neurotransmitters governed this blocked response? Norbert Matussek and his group at the University of Munich used amphetamine as a challenge to answer this question. In the 1960s, Matussek, like an entire generation of neuroscientists, had studied with Bernard Brodie at the National Heart Institute (part of NIH). Back in Munich and working under the chief of the service, Hanns Hippius, Matussek was intent upon using neuroendocrine methods to study brain function. In 1976, his group found the GH response to amphetamine blunted in patients with endogenous depression, but not in those with reactive depression or in normal subjects. "Our findings are consistent with the norepinephrine functional deficiency hypothesis for a subgroup of depressive disorders," the investigators wrote.[37] What receptors were involved, presynaptic or postsynaptic? Matussek used clonidine, a postsynaptic receptor agonist, to stimulate growth hormone secretion, and then observed the difference in depressives and controls. Matussek later recalled the circumstances of the research:

> Obviously the clonidine-GH stimulation test had to be first investigated in untreated, depressed patients. These are however admitted very seldom to our clinic and thus are like rare jewels. Collaboration with H. Schultes, an extraordinary and cooperative psychiatrist with a great ambulance [outpatient service] in the Danube valley, helped us in this respect.... Every Sunday afternoon, one or two of us went 300 km by car first to drink some good Wachauian wine on a Sunday night and to look for untreated, depressed patients in Schultes's ambulance at 7 A.M. on Monday morning.

In 1977, the group reported at the Sixth World Congress of Psychiatry in Hawaii that "the GH response to clonidine was blunted in endogenous depressive patients, but not in non-endogenous depressed patients and controls; we interpreted our results as being evidence of a subsensitivity of postsynaptic alpha-adrenoceptors...." These studies, together with data from other investigators, "gave good evidence for the hypothesis of postsynaptic changes of the alpha-adre-noceptor sensitivity as a possible neurobiological defect in depression."[38] (Alpha-adrenoceptors are found in the brain and respond to stimulation by norepinephrine [noradrenaline]; these findings buttressed a "nora-drenergic" hypothesis of depression.)

The subsequent skepticism about these one-neurotransmitter-to-one-disease hypotheses does not diminish the magnitude of these pioneering efforts. Using a new technique, RIA, these investigators were truly opening a window into the brain's hypothalamus. In 1976, at an annual meeting of the American College of Neuropsychopharmacology, Bernard Carroll said of the knowledge that RIA had pried free: "The research designs in clinical psychoneuroendocrinology reflect this 'neuroendocrine window' strategy: we no longer simply measure base-line levels of hormones in urine or blood but [with RIA techniques gain] information about the integrity of limbic-hypothalamic interactions, and thus about the function of the limbic system itself in psychopathological states, or in response to psychotropic drugs."[39]

RIAs are science. But in the hands of the peptide enthusiasts, the whole approach to psychiatric illness via these tiny releasing factors might press biological reductionism to its limits. Veteran members of the American College of Neuropsychopharmacology remember scratching their heads in the 1980s, unable to understand what relationship these chemicals had to illness in humans. A rather jaundiced Jean Rossier, a French neuroscientist who had joined Guillemin and Floyd Bloom at the Salk Institute in San Diego in the late 1970s, said, "The idea that one peptide could control one behavior was so widespread at the end of the seventies that biological psychiatrists proposed that the cause of many psychiatric diseases could be a marked increase of a particular peptide." He added sarcastically, "If this hypothesis was right, therapy of psychiatric disease could be performed by dialysis to wash out the excess peptide that was supposed to be accumulating in the blood."[40]

This new peptide lore played out clinically first in the thyroid axis.

Thyroid at the University of North Carolina

The signaling that takes place in depression along the hypothalamic-pituitary-thyroid (HPT) axis is comparable to that along the HPA axis. Both constitute fundamental evidence that in melancholia, mania, and other serious mental disorders, the neuroendocrine system is disordered.

In the late 1960s, Peter Whybrow, who had just graduated in medicine in England, went to the UNC for training in its newly established department of psychiatry. He later wrote, "During the late 1960s UNC was on the cusp of the biological revolution that was beginning in American psychiatry." The department chair, the Scotsman John Ewing, was willing to accept "foreign nationals," and Whybrow came on board, to learn from such figures as Art Prange and Frank Kane and to study alongside such fellow residents as Fred Goodwin and Joe Mendels.[41]

The key figure in thyroid at UNC was Arthur Prange, born in Grand Rapids, Michigan, in 1926. Prange earned a medical degree in 1950 from the University of Michigan and trained in anesthesiology in Detroit the following year. After serving as chief of anesthesiology at the U.S. Naval Hospital in Key West, Florida, in 1952–1953, Prange decided that psychiatry better suited his interests, and in 1954 began training in psychiatry at the UNC; he was to remain there for the rest of his career.[42] Psychiatry, as noted, was just beginning at UNC, and Prange was in the first class of trainees.

Prange's neuroendocrine interests dated back to 1960, when he learned of a depressed patient of Frank Kane's who'd been treated with the tricyclic antidepressant drug imipramine and "excess amounts of desiccated thyroid as replacement medication." As a result, the patient "was experiencing runs of paroxysmal auricular tachycardia" (episodes of accelerated heartbeat). Prange mentioned this excess-thyroid patient to Morris Lipton, a biologically oriented staff member and graduate of the University of Chicago who had joined the department at UNC in 1959 as director of research (and led the department from 1970 to 1973). Morrie Lipton had worked at the Michael Reese Hospital in Chicago and was sensitive to endocrine issues. Indeed, Lipton is often seen as having "opened up the peptides."[43] Lipton advised Prange "to study this patient and, having studied her, to stay with the various facets of research that her case suggested." Prange added, "I have done so."[44]

Under the benevolent gaze of Lipton, Prange made the department of psychiatry at UNC a world center of thyroid psychiatry. In 1968 the group recruited the neuropharmacologist George Breese from the NIH. Prange went up to Bethesda for four months to work in the laboratory of Irwin Kopin, who was director of the NIMH Intramural program, becoming closely associated with such internationally known figures as Seymour Kety and Julius Axelrod. Upon his return, Prange organized a clinical research program at the Dorothea Dix Hospital, thirty miles from Chapel Hill.

Their research concerned mainly the use of L-triiodothyronine (T_3) to augment the benefits of imipramine in depression. At the annual meeting of the APA in Boston in May of 1968 and in the *American Journal of Psychiatry* in 1969, Prange reported, "Imipramine may elevate effective biogenic concentration, while T_3 increases receptor sensitivity."[45] (A more definitive trial forty years later, in 2008, led by Michael Posternak at the Massachusetts General Hospital, with Prange as co-investigator, found that "the likelihood of experiencing a positive response at any point over the 6 wk trial was 4.5 times greater in the adjunctive T3 cohort . . ." than in the placebo cohort.[46])

Lipton encouraged Prange to spend 1968–1969 as a visiting scientist with Alec Coppen at the Medical Research Council Unit at West Park Hospital in Epsom, England, to study serotonin, on which Coppen was then a world authority. Prange saw these new neurotransmitter theories of depression as a "'competing' body of knowledge." He was joined by Peter Whybrow, the young English psychiatrist who had trained as a resident at UNC. Prange said, "Coppen, Whybrow and I performed a major clinical trial with L-tryptophan, the precursor of the indoleamine neurotransmitter serotonin, in depressed patients. We found that it was about as effective an antidepressant as imipramine." T_3, they noted, enhanced the action of imipramine but not that of L-tryptophan.[47] This supported a hypothesis of "thyroid catecholamine-receptor interaction."[48] (Imipramine acts preferentially on norepinephrine, a catecholamine neurotransmitter.) Coppen had made the surprising claim that L-tryptophan was as effective as ECT in depression.[49] This claim was dismissed in 1970 by Bernard Carroll, Brian Davies, and Robert Mowbray in Melbourne, who studied the two treatments head to head, rather than relying on historical data to compare them as Coppen had done.[50])

In 1971, Prange's group studied the hypothalamic releasing factor TRH, the structure of which Guillemin and Schally had just described in 1969. Might it have an antidepressant effect? Indeed, Prange and co-workers found in 1972 that a sample of depressed patients experienced brief relief from a single injection of TRH. Yet the following year, 1973, the Neuropharmacology Advisory Committee of the FDA concluded that evidence for TRH as an antidepressant was not encouraging.[51]

But Prange had a more important finding about TRH, destined to become a durable result in biological psychiatry: that the TSH response to TRH was blunted (TSH is from the anterior pituitary). Depression is marked by "hypothalamic underactivity." Prange presented the preliminary findings at a meeting of the Collegium Internationale Neuro-Psychopharmacologicum (CINP) in Copenhagen in August 1972 and then published a definitive version in the *Lancet* three months later.[52] What Sachar reported for GH, the Prange group now discovered for the thyroid hormones. As Prange later observed, this finding of a "grossly deficient" TSH response to exogenous TRH "has become one of the most widely replicated findings in biological psychiatry."[53] Prange later called it "an endocrine scar."[54] (Like the DST, the TRH–TSH test also predicted relapse in depressive illness, in this case, after convulsive therapy.[55])

Among the scholars trained by the Prange group was Charles Nemeroff, later chair of psychiatry at Emory University in Atlanta. Nemeroff graduated in medicine from UNC in 1981 and finished his psychiatry training there in 1983, going on to earn a Ph.D. in pharmacology. In 1977, still a medical student, Nemeroff led the Prange group in the study of neurotensin, a broadly distributed peptide, found also in the gut, that affected central nervous function.[56] He continued this work after moving to Duke in 1983. The list of psychoactive hypothalamic peptides grew.

The clinical results for TRH treatment were disappointing. There seemed to be a subgroup of severely ill depressives, as Wayne Furlong at the University of Toronto reported in 1976, who responded to TRH, though the responsive population was poorly characterized (they also responded well to ECT).[57] But on the whole, as Prange, Nemeroff, and Lipton pointed out at an ACNP meeting in 1978, TRH aggravated paranoia, while offering some benefit in the negative symptoms of schizophrenia. Interestingly, the authors said, "Since TRH may have prodopaminergic properties, these findings call into question the relevance of the DA [dopamine] hypothesis for some subgroups of schizophrenia patients."[58] This conclusion was of special note because, by the late 1970s, the one-neurotransmitter-one-disease theory had been elevated to gospel, and blocking dopamine receptors was seen as the key to the action of antipsychotics. (Much later, in 2005, Peter Whybrow, now chair of the department of psychiatry at the Neuropsychiatric Institute of Los Angeles, and colleagues at other institutions did find evidence of the therapeutic effectiveness of TRH in bipolar depression, given intravenously at midnight, "when the circadian sensitivity of the TRH receptor is at its peak."[59])

In 1982, Prange and Peter Loosen, a medical graduate in 1970 of the University of Munich who had trained at UNC and was currently on staff, put the TRH test on the map as a second possible neuroendocrine marker of depression: a sluggish TSH response to TRH meant "a defect in the central regulation of the pituitary-thyroid axis."[60] As Alan Levy and Stephen Stern, in the mood disorders program at Ohio State University, noted in 1987 in a study of twenty-nine depressed hospitalized patients, both the DST and the TRH-stimulation test "significantly discriminated patients with non-endogenous depression from those with endogenous depression."[61] This overlap in the two tests, Bernard Carroll said, "introduces the possibility of a test battery or sequential testing that would in principle outperform any single test."[62]

Twenty to thirty percent of patients with mood disorders show some abnormality of the HPT system.[63] In the 1980s, attention turned to the possible behavioral effects of hypothyroidism, a matter long of interest in endocrine psychiatry but now under the magnifying glass of TRH testing. In 1981, Mark Gold and colleagues at Fair Oaks Hospital in Summit, New Jersey, found that among 250 consecutive patients referred for depression or anergia, 20 had some degree of hypothyroidism. The authors counseled, "All patients with a poor response to traditional psychiatric treatments for depression and anergia should have a comprehensive thyroid evaluation."[64] (This rate of hypothyroidism in a psychiatric population was low: among medication treatment-failures with depression at the Western Psychiatric Institute in Pittsburgh, fully half had subclinical hypothyroidism.[65] Florian Holsboer in Munich, an international authority, considers this rate of HPT abnormality of great importance.[66])

The question of hypothyroidism—"fraught with clinical significance" as Prange put it[67]—captured the attention of the UNC group. Frederick Goodwin had trained in psychiatry at UNC, going on in 1965 to intramural research at NIMH. In 1983, as director of intramural research, he and colleagues discovered overt hypothyroidism in fully half of the rapid-cycling bipolar patients at NIH's Clinical Center—and in none of the non–rapid-cycling group. Furthermore, 92 percent of the rapid-cyclers had elevated TSH levels, versus only 32 percent of the non-rapid-cyclers.[68] These dramatic findings explained the efficacy that Rolf Gjessing found before the Second World War in treating "periodic catatonia" with thyroid preparations.[69]

Adding thyroxine (T4) to the basic medication—mainly lithium—of the rapid-cyclers who had been treatment-resistant proved highly effective, as Peter Whybrow and a colleague reported in 1990.[70] As well, successful treatment with antidepressants reduced thyroid levels. In 1984, Russell Joffe of the University of Toronto—together with colleagues at NIMH, where he was a fellow—suggested that "a decrease, rather than an increase, in thyroid indices is associated with an acute treatment response in affective illness," upending the previous conventional wisdom.[71] (In 1993, Peter Loosen's team, now at Vanderbilt, confirmed that "[a] significant proportion of the sample [26%] showed some abnormality in thyroid hormone levels.... The majority of these returned to normal with antidepressant therapy."[72] Thus, giving thyroid improved depression; and giving antidepressants improved the thyroid picture. The HPT axis clearly was intertwined with depressive illness.

But "intertwined" is a metaphor, not a diagram. The relationship between the thyroid hormones and mental disease remained anything but clear. There is a non sequitur, or an apparent conundrum, in the above data. As Carroll puts it, "On one hand, giving T4 supplements improves the response to antidepressant drugs. That suggests the thyroid system was a quart low. On the other hand, antidepressant drugs reduce thyroid hormone production. That suggests the thyroid system was a bit overactive to begin with."[73]

We ran this conundrum past Joffe, who in 2007 was professor of psychiatry at the New Jersey Medical School. His interesting response, really a comment on the opaque nature of a number of neuroendocrine findings, merits sharing:

Joffe wrote,[74] and we quote at length:

This is a very complex issue. To summarize:

T4 has been described as an adjunctive mood stabilizer in bipolar subjects, especially rapid cyclers, usually at high doses. The data to support this are quite limited with minimal controlled data. This is a long-term maintenance effect.

Short-term antidepressant treatment causes significant but limited decreases in T4. These decreases are practically never outside the normal range for T4. The pathophysiological significance is of unknown certainty. It may be that:

1. Limited decreases in T4 are required for treatment response.
2. The decreases reflect an iodinase deficiency.
3. The decreases occur to normalize a compensatory increase in thyroid hormones which occurs in response to depression.
4. Another unknown reason.

The issue is further complicated by the fact that we do not know what or if there is a primary thyroid defect in depression or bipolar disorder. Moreover, these are all plasma measures and it is unclear to what extent they reflect brain thyroid function as the brain handles thyroid hormone differently from other organs and tissues.

Perhaps the greater paradox is that lithium is a mood stabilizer and decreases thyroid function.

I am sure this does not clarify things that well but it is the state of the field. Unlike the adrenal axis, the thyroid is implicated in depression and bipolar illness but the relationship is complex. T4 may be a mood stabilizer but this is still definitively to be shown; changes in thyroid hormones accompany changes in mood state.

The authors add that this may be another example of the confusion engendered by the separation of unipolar major depression and bipolar disorder. Dr. Joffe continues: "The pathophysiological significance of all of this is uncertain and a specific pathology of the thyroid axis in mood disorders has not been identified. This is a complex issue which still puzzles (and frustrates) me after 20 years of study."

Prange mused about these paradoxical findings in 1998: "Like lithium, T_3 as an adjunct will convert approximately two-thirds of antidepressant drug failures to successes.... That an antithyroid drug like lithium and a prothyroid substance like T_3 accomplishes nearly the same goal in *most* members of a population begs for research."[75]

In Florence in 1991 at the World Congress of Biological Psychiatry, Prange briefly met Lithuanian psychiatrist and endocrinologist Robertas Bunevicius. They began a correspondence, and in 1997, Bunevicius won a Fulbright Award to spend six months at Chapel Hill.[76] Bunevicius and Prange puzzled over data on thyroid supplementation in nonpsychiatric patients with hypothyroidism in Kaunas, Lithuania. They concluded in 1999 in the *New England Journal of Medicine* that, "In patients with hypothyroidism, partial substitution of triiodothyronine [T_3] for thyroxine [T_4] may improve mood and neuropsychological function." Thus, natural T_3 might have a specific cognitive and mood effect.[76]

A signal accomplishment was seeing TRH in its commanding role as a prime mover, alongside CRH among the hypothalamic peptides, directing not just the synthesis of thyroid hormones but regulating the "general TRH homeostatic system." Its components included the entire hypothalamic-pituitary neuroendocrine system; the "brainstem/mid-brain/spinal cord system"; the limbic-cortical system; and the "chronobiological system." This overarching concept, published in 2003, should have given TRH a place of honor in therapeutics.[77] Unfortunately, it did not.

Prange, near the end of his scholarly career, noted that this research "brought me nearly full circle." (He had started his career in anesthesiology and fled it for psychiatry.) "Life may or may not be short, but the art is surely long," he said.[78]

Florian Holsboer and the Max Planck Institute in Munich

After a gap of many years, interest in CRH and cortisol shifted to Germany, where Florian Holsboer in Munich again picked up the torch. Holsboer grew up in Munich and completed a Ph.D. in chemistry at the Ludwig-Maximilians-University in 1975, graduating in medicine four years later. He trained in psychiatry in Munich under Hanns Hippius and in Mainz under Otto Benkert, completing his postgraduate thesis in 1984. In 1987, he became chair of the department of psychiatry at the University of Freiburg and in 1989 director of the Max Planck Institute of Psychiatry in Munich, a research institute that Emil Kraepelin founded in 1917.

His entry into psychiatry from chemistry is interesting, giving him an innovative view of "biological." Rather than starting with disordered behavior and attempting to find biological explanations for it, Holsboer started with the biology and proceeded, as is common in clinical medicine, to the identification of disease entities by signs and symptoms, verification by laboratory tests, and validation by treatment response. This puts him much closer to Samuel Guze's "medical model" of psychiatry[80] than to a psychiatry limiting itself to verbally transmitted information.

The progress of Holsboer's work in Mainz and Munich—and the controversy it elicited—reflects the difficulty in putting the basic science of neuroendocrinology into clinical application: At the end of the day, the discoveries rest on a firm platform of neuroscience, but what do they mean?

Holsboer debuted his scientific career on a doubting note: the DST did not seem terribly useful in the diagnosis of endogenous depression. In a 1980 study in Munich, he and colleagues discovered that the frequency of cortisol nonsuppression after dexamethasone was only around 20 to 30 percent, depending on whether the ICD, Newcastle, or Research Diagnostic Criteria scales were used to diagnose "endogenous" depression. Nonetheless, the endogenous depression scores were higher than those for "neurotic/reactive depression" and "schizophrenia/schizoaffective."[81]

This tepid finding produced a vigorous response from Carroll, with whom Holsboer was to cross swords continually over the years about diagnostic markers in depression. Carroll said that the Munich results were entirely atypical of the solid findings about "the predictive values of an abnormal DST result for endogenous depression," which Carroll put at 93 percent. Furthermore, Holsboer's findings, Carroll said, suggested that the diagnosis of depression in Munich was probably not quite up to snuff: "This may serve as a signal that their diagnostic practice differs from that of most other workers. As more groups begin to use the DST we may expect that a consensus about its diagnostic value in psychiatry will emerge. All we can say for the present is that we are moving towards a redefinition of endogenous depression," one involving new biological markers that might well trump the "traditional clinical features."[82] Carroll's critique strikes us as reasonable: There may well have been several different types of depression in the Munich clinical population; for example, psychotic depression or schizoaffective. The question here is not why only 20 to 30 percent of a heterogeneous, newly admitted sample were nonsuppressors, but what is common to that 20 to 30 percent?

In the next several years, Holsboer's work centered more on the DST as a marker of recovery—and on persistently positive DSTs as a marker of persistent illness. "The most important observation," he wrote in 1982, "is that in all cases normalization of the HPA activity precedes clinical recovery. Furthermore a patient who appears to be clinically appropriate for discharge and fails to suppress cortisol after dexamethasone has a high risk for relapse."[83]

From late 1982 on at Mainz, Holsboer's interest turned toward CRH. In research published in 1984, the Holsboer group injected sixteen unmedicated depressed patients with CRH. Both cortisol and ACTH levels rose. The investigators concluded that increased HPA function in depression was not the result of hypersensitivity of the pituitary or the adrenal cortex but that "[a] limbic-hypothalamic overactivity is more likely to be the mechanism underlying hypercortisolism associated with depression."[84] This was a significant finding.

But what endocrine findings were distinctive in depression? Later in 1984, the Holsboer group at Mainz administered CRH to twelve depressed patients and nine healthy controls. In depressed patients and controls, cortisol and ACTH levels rose, but in depressed patients the ACTH levels did not rise as much: the ACTH response to CRH was "blunted" while the cortisol response was not.[85] Something about the HPA axis in depression meant that its responses—at a "suprapituitary" site—to such a probe were deficient.

Simultaneously, Charles Nemeroff at Duke University was finding high CRH levels in the cerebrospinal fluid of depressed patients.[86] (In 1999, Holsboer argued for "CRH hyperactivity in depression."[87])

Nemeroff and associates also learned that CRF could be manipulated in such a way as to reproduce a depressive syndrome. As David Rubinow, at the time at NIMH, summarized this work, "You can manipulate CRF in such a way as to reproduce the [depressive] syndrome . . . . There are animal studies showing that you can create a depressive-like syndrome with CRF, you can produce antidepressant effects by knocking out CRF."[88] The hormone that stimulated the HPA axis thus seemed to be implicated in depression. But how?

What about pretreating depressed patients with dexamethasone and then administering CRH? This caused cortisol to surge. Holsboer in 1986 noted, "In contrast to normal controls, depressed patients pre-treated with dexamethasone responded to CRH with increased cortisol release." As the patients recovered, CRH slowly failed to elicit these rushes of cortisol.[89] At the conference where Holsboer presented these findings, Nemeroff was chair of the session. This marked the beginning of a lifelong friendship between the two investigators. This was also the beginning of the combined DEX/CRH test for which Holsboer became well known.

Was the blunted ACTH response (but normal cortisol response) to exogenous CRH specific to depression? Apparently not. In 1987, the Holsboer group at Mainz discovered the same finding in panic disorder and alcoholism. "In these diseases, enhanced baseline pituitary adreno-cortical activity appears to be driven by a CNS disturbance resulting in overactive CRH secreting neurons."[90] The paper was dedicated to Jules Angst, director of research at the Zurich University Psychiatric Hospital and pioneer in psychopharmacology, whom Holsboer considered to be a mentor.

Giving patients CRH after pretreating them with dexametha-sone, is this not really just the equivalent of the dexamethasone sup-pression test? No, said Holsboer, it is not. In 1987 he determined that, even if depressed patients were pretreated with dexamethasone, administering CRH resulted in further releases of ACTH and cortisol. This did not occur in normal controls, as Holsboer's collaborator Ulrich von Bardeleben had demonstrated in 1985.[91] In theory, further increases in ACTH and cortisol after exogenous CRH should not happen: Dexamethasone would keep the glucocorticoid feedback signal high, so CRH should not be able to boost ACTH or cortisol still higher. Dexamethasone had apparently not entirely knocked out the capacity of the HPA axis to still respond to other agents, and CRH was a potent challenge. The ability of CRH to stimulate further release of cortisol and ACTH disappeared as the patients' depression started to clear.

Finally—and perhaps most interestingly—the "DST/CRH" test functioned in depressed patients independently of whether they were otherwise dexamethasone suppressors or nonsuppressors.[92] Holsboer's test clearly reflected something different than did Barney Carroll's DST. Thus, Holsboer's DST/CRH test sounded very much like a biological marker of what he would soon call "dysfunction" of the HPA axis.

The first airing of Holsboer's "combined dexamethasone/human-CRH challenge test" for an international audience took place in 1989 at the University of Freiburg, where Holsboer had in the meantime become head of the department of psychiatry.[93] (Holsboer had published a report in German in 1988.[94]) Holsboer and Bardeleben administered a "combined dexamethasone–human corticotrophin-releasing hormone (hCRH) challenge test" to fourteen depressed patients and fourteen controls. After pretreating the patients with dexamethasone the day before, they administered CRH, then drew blood samples at periodic intervals for several hours thereafter. A multiple regression analysis revealed that age and severity of depression influenced cortisol secretion in the depressed patients but not in the controls. (Also, vasopressin seemed to play a role in the escape from suppression among the depressed patients but not among the controls.)

The clinical launch took place at the department of psychiatry of the University of Basel and was led by Edith Holsboer-Trachsler. She and her group administered human CRH to fourteen depressed patients who had been pretreated with dexamethasone and to thirteen controls. The depressed patients had cortisol and ACTH responses significantly higher than those of the controls. Moreover, as soon as the depressed patients were treated with the tricyclic antidepressant trimipramine, their plasma cortisol normalized (though "ACTH release remained exaggerated"). The authors concluded that the test "may be of particular value in the detection of state-dependent changes of pituitary-adrenocortical neuroregulation."[95]

Was the sensitivity of the "DEX/CRH" test, in the hands of Holsboer's group at the Max Planck Institute of Psychiatry in Munich where Holsboer had just become director, greater than that of Carroll's DST? Yes, they asserted. In 1994, in research led by Isabella Heuser, the Max Planck team concluded, "The sensitivity of the DEX/CRH test for MDE [major depressive episode] (about 80%) greatly exceeds that of the standard DST (1 mg–2 mg of DEX), which has been reported to average about 44% in a meta-analysis of the literature data: in our sample the sensitivity of the DST was about 25%."[96]

Carroll and Holsboer

In the interests of a meaningful scientific exchange, we asked Carroll to comment on the Holsboer DEX/CRH test. Carroll said:

> The Holsboer group generally gloss over the problem of low specificity for the DEX-CRH test. They have not demonstrated that the trade-off between higher sensitivity and lower specificity compared with the original DST is a net plus. In some contexts it may be a net plus but in other contexts the lower specificity will be a liability. As for the speculation about vasopressin secretion, they never tested depressed patients with CRH plus vasopressin. That would have been a necessary control. They also never excluded low dexamethasone levels as a cause of the increased ACTH/cortisol after CRH administration. Low dexamethasone levels are an important confound in both the DST and the DEX-CRH test. Holsboer has some speculation about the "early biophase" that leads him to ignore ambient dexamethasone levels at the time the CRH is given in his combined test. The evidence is to the contrary, however.[97]

Unlike Carroll's view of the DST, Holsboer did not consider his own test to be a marker of melancholia. Instead, the Holsboer group said in 1994, "The DEX/CRH-test phenomenon constitutes a neuroendocrine sign of . . . various disorders and emphasizes the usefulness of the DEX/CRH test to monitor the course of these disorders."[98]

Carroll responds:

> What exactly is the DEX-CRH test a marker for? For that matter, what is the end point of this test? Is it ACTH response or cortisol response? Holsboer's group vacillates on this issue. What exactly does the DEX-CRH test test? And does the DEX-CRH test with ACTH as the dependent variable test the same thing as the DEX-CRH test with cortisol as the dependent variable? Holsboer is quite indefinite on these fundamental issues. The usual formulation from Holsboer's group is that

abnormal DEX-CRH test results signify "impaired HPA regulation" or "dysregulated HPA function." What does that tell a clinician? Where is the methodological standardization of variables like dexamethasone dosage or plasma dexamethasone concentration windows or blood sampling frequency? It is clear in Holsboer's own data that the DST part of the DEX-CRH test predicts the CRH part (cortisol response to CRH) in depressed patients.[99] This makes it likely that a dexamethasone concentration confound needs to be ruled out in published studies of the DEX-CRH test, just as for the DST.

The interpretive problem is that the DEX-CRH test does not necessarily indicate baseline "hyperactivity" of the HPA axis but simply hyper-responsiveness to administered CRH in non-physiologic dosing. The response time course of ACTH and cortisol in the DEX-CRH test, or in the CRH test for that matter, bears no resemblance to anything seen in normal HPA physiology except maybe provocative procedures like the insulin tolerance test. Again, what exactly does the test test? It cannot tell us anything about what is going on in the brain. It tests only pituitary and adrenal responsiveness to one secretagogue for ACTH. Holsboer and colleagues have never given a sustained account of why test responses are blunted [in depression] without DEX but exaggerated after DEX. The parsimonious explanation is that baseline CRH test responses are blunted because of the high ambient cortisol in the depressed patients, whereas after DEX the responses are exaggerated because of low DEX levels in comparison to controls. This interpretation accords with the endocrine facts, whereas the metaphysical expression "HPA axis dysregulation" is too vague to be of any use."[100]

In his own work, Carroll invoked a much more precise mechanism: "an abnormal limbic system drive on the HPA axis in primary depressive illness."[101]

Yet Holsboer's DEX/CRH test has found friends. Christine Heim and Charles Nemeroff at Emory University, for example, used the DEX-CRH test on men with major depression to highlight the role of childhood trauma, a role apparently more difficult to discern with the DST alone.[102]

David Rubinow believes that the discovery of CRF justly helped pitch the dexamethasone test into disuse. "With the development of

CRF and the understanding of the axis, suddenly they had a much more elegant way of being able to explore the axis than dexamethasone."

Do you think it's superior to the DST? asked an interviewer.

"The people who have spent the most time on this, that I know, are Charlie [Nemeroff] and Florian [Holsboer], and they say that it is much better at distinguishing a normal response from an abnormal response. That's what they say."[103]

So the jury is still out on Holsboer's test.

The Munich Group Goes Beyond the Test

There was yet another area where the Holsboer group opened up new avenues: neuroactive steroids, which alter neuronal excitability or affect gene expression. Rubinow commented, "As soon as people leave medical school they forget everything they ever learned about reproductive endocrinology.... [Holsboer's] work with neurosteroids is very, very important, and not as widely attended to, because people aren't familiar with them."[104] In a collaboration with Rainer Rupprecht going back to 1993, Holsboer's group looked at the action of neurosteroids on different receptors.[105] By 1998 they were studying the effects in depression of agents such as fluoxetine on various forms of progesterone in the brain: "These results provide the first clinical evidence of a possible role of neuroactive steroids in successful antidepressant therapy."[106] This was a significant step in moving the dialogue beyond the conventional "biogenic amine" neurotransmitters.

Finally, the 1970s and 1980s were full of buzz about receptor binding, and it is appropriate to mention the Munich group's contribution of the "corticosteroid receptor hypothesis of depression." In 1969, Bruce McEwen and associates at Rockefeller University found that various limbic structures in rat brain retained corticosterone, without the mechanism's being evident.[107] In 1973, Bernard Grosser and colleagues at the University of Utah showed that macromolecules within cells had a high affinity for radiotagged corticosteroids.[108] Three years later, in 1976, the McEwen group found a difference in the binding of such steroids from one area of the brain to another and speculated that they might be due to "the presence of various kinds of receptor molecules."[109] This led to much research on the binding of glucocorticoids in the brain as a possible mechanism in depression, which will not be reviewed here. In 2000, Holsboer suggested that "impaired GR [corticosteroid receptor] signalling is a key mechanism in the pathogenesis of depression." The research of the Munich group in mouse genetics, Holsboer argued, buttressed this hypothesis.[110] At the present writing, the interaction between genetics and corticosteroid receptor signalling in depression has not become clearer—though it remains an active initiative in endocrine psychiatry.

Drugs

Until the 1980s, the prospects of treating melancholia with drugs, especially its psychotic version, had not been rosy. The tricyclic antidepressants were famously ineffective in psychotic depression, and combination treatments of antidepressants and antipsychotics had limited efficacy.[111] Electroconvulsive therapy was a much more certain remedy, but many patients and their families shied away from "shock treatment."

Previous researchers had some results with the hypothalamic releasing factors, but more as probes than as therapies. In 1976, Robert Rubin, at the Harbor General Hospital Campus in Torrance, California, using RIA, found that in normal men the antipsychotic drug haloperidol increased the pituitary hormone prolactin, while having no effect on the gonadotropins or on GH.[112] This was a more sophisticated version of an assay Sachar had attempted several years earlier. As Rubin put it, the research was "establishing the prolactin response as one measure of the potency of dopamine-blocking antipsychotic drugs."[113]

Into this relative vacuum now rushed several young researchers. This story begins in 1982 as two staffers at McLean Hospital in Belmont, Massachusetts—Alan Schatzberg and Anthony Rothschild—began, under the guidance of Jonathan Cole, studies of dexamethasone and neurotransmitters. Schatzberg, thirty-eight at the time, had just become chief of the service; Rothschild, twenty-nine, was a clinical fellow. They found the dexamethasone suppression test differentiated psychotic depression in a population of psychiatric patients. "Our data seem to indicate," they wrote, "a trend towards higher postdexamethasone cortisol levels in unipolar psychotic depressives as compared to bipolar psychotic depressives.... There may be a subgroup of psychotic patients with unipolar depression with very high cortisol levels and another subgroup with lower levels."[114] Thus, the authors confirmed Carroll's finding in 1976 of a biological marker for psychotic depression.[115] There had also been previous findings of psychosis in Cushing disease. So, the idea that high cortisol levels might lead to psychosis was not new.

Schatzberg and Rothschild's contribution, however, was to propose that cortisol might lead to psychosis through a dopamine mechanism. In 1984, they found that dexamethasone raised plasma dopamine levels, a possible explanation of psychiatric disturbances in patients on steroid treatment. In a bit of a leap from the paper's main finding, they mused, "Indeed, it is interesting to speculate as to whether cortisol-induced increases in free dopamine within the central nervous system could result in the eventual expression of psychotic symptomatology in the depressed patient."[116] In 1985 they found that the glucocorticoids enhanced dopamine activity in the rat brain, suggesting this as the mechanism of psychosis in depression.[117]

Over the next several years, Rothschild and Schatzberg reported "cortisol-induced increases in dopamine [that] may play an important role in the pathogenesis of delusional symptoms in depressed... patients," as they said in 1988. Logical treatment strategies were either to interfere with cortisol synthesis or to use "specific glucocorticoid receptor blockers" to reduce plasma cortisol. Dexamethasone could block cortisol synthesis (for DST suppressors) but would not reduce dopamine. They used ketoconazole and metyrapone, inhibitors of steroid biosynthesis, to disrupt the secretion of cortisol, with limited benefit. No drugs were as yet available in psychiatry for blocking the cortisol receptors.[118] (This would later be the role of mifepristone; ketoconazole is an antifungal triazole;[119] metyrapone is a propanone; both were later tested without convincing results as antidepressants.)

Now the scene shifts from McLean Hospital to Montreal, birthplace of neuroendocrinology, where neuroendocrinologist Beverley Murphy, director of the Reproductive Physiology Unit at the Montreal General Hospital and consultant in psychiatry at the Royal Victoria Hospital, had become an important figure. In the late 1960s, she described a highly specific method of measuring cortisol involving competitive protein binding—research that later became a citation classic.[120] She writes, in a memoir requested by the authors, "In the early 1980s I became interested in the psychiatric aspects of endocrinology because hypercortisolemia had been shown to be the most clearcut biochemical abnormality of major depression and that many patients were resistant to its suppression by dexamethasone."[121] She continues:

At that time—March, 1988—I was interested in studying hormone changes in the premenstrual syndrome and thought it would be of interest to compare these patients with women suffering from major depression. Due to space constraints in the Montreal General Hospital, I was using some laboratory space of a friend of mine, Dr. Marion Birmingham, a steroid chemist who carried out her research in the Department of Psychiatry at the Allan Memorial Institute of the Royal Victoria Hospital, so I got to know some of the local psychiatrists. A student was dispatched to the inpatient psychiatric ward to find a suitable patient. He found a 31-year-old woman who had been admitted several times over the previous 9 months for suicidal attempts and in whom several antidepressants had been ineffective. On examination she was thin, had low normal blood pressure and was obviously very depressed. Much to my surprise, her plasma cortisol levels were over 30 µg/100 ml (1500 nmol/L), showed little diurnal variation, and did not suppress with dexamethasone. Biochemically she had Cushing's syndrome, but physically she showed no signs of it. Her electrolytes, abdominal ultrasound, and brain CT scan were entirely normal. Since her treating psychiatrist was at a loss as to how to treat her, I suggested that we try to lower her cortisol levels, using the same drugs for a "medical adrenalectomy" in Cushing's syndrome. He agreed and she was given aminoglutethimide 250 mg bid along with 20 mg cortisol to ensure that the cortisol levels would not drop too low ["bid" means twice daily; aminoglutethimide is an adrenal steroidogenesis blocker, once indicated as an antiepileptic]. On the third day of treatment she reported that her mind "felt clear for the first time in months" and that she had more energy. The dose was increased to tid [three times daily] and then to qid [four times daily]. Metyrapone was also used briefly. After 8 weeks of treatment with steady improvement, mainly as an out-patient, the drugs were gradually withdrawn and she remained well. I last heard from her a few years ago and she was still well, on no treatment, and had never had a recurrence of her depression.[122]

It is possible that Murphy had excellent results in a single case for unknown reasons (possibly by suppressing kindled seizure activity in the patient's limbic system). We know now that when drugs like aminoglutethimide or metyrapone are given chronically to patients with a functioning pituitary gland, they lead to massive increases of ACTH, which soon causes breakthrough of the inhibition of cortisol synthesis. In clinical endocrinology, such drugs are useful primarily in patients with non-ACTH-dependent Cushing disease, such as an adrenal adenoma or carcinoma. There is, in the view of some authorities, no reason to consider that adrenal corticosteroid synthesis inhibitors would be useful in treating depressed patients whose pituitary glands are functional.[123]

Nonetheless, in 1991, Murphy noted the clinical similarities between major depression and the depression of Cushing's syndrome. She hypothesized that a derangement in the body's steroid system might be driving the depression, which itself had originated in the brain. "Steroid suppressive agents may also alleviate endogenous depression."[124]

At this time, Murphy and her collaborators completed a small, uncontrolled trial of steroid suppression in major depression, using aminoglutethimide, ketoconazole, and metyrapone—roughly the drugs the McLean group had been using for several years—as suppressants. Of the ten patients in the trial, eight completed the study and six responded well, two partially.[125] This was proof of concept. (Rothschild and Schatzberg were vexed that Murphy cited virtually none of the previous research on steroids and depression, including their own; she responded rather sovereignly that she had been studying drugs in depression that inhibit steroid biosythesis while others had merely studied the administration of steroids in the treatment of psychosis, not depression.[126])

Two years later, in 1993, Murphy and collaborators at McGill University gave four patients with "chronic severe depression" a new steroid synthesized in France in 1980 by Roussel-Uclaf, a French subsidiary of the German company Hoechst, called RU-486 (mifepristone). In low doses mifepristone was an abortifacient (and a subject of great controversy at the FDA over its licensing in the United States). In high doses, it was hoped that, as an antiglucocorticoid, it might be an antidepressant by suppressing the release of cortisol. This was not the first report of mifepristone's psychiatric effect,[127] but it was the first trial. Just as the trial came to an end, the politics of mifepristone exploded and the suppliers canceled the drug, making further research impossible.[128]

By 1995, Murphy and collaborators had used aminoglutethimide, metyrapone, and ketoconazole on twenty patients suffering from treatment-resistant depression. Even if small, the results are impressive. Of the eight psychotic depressives who completed treatment, five responded completely; of the nine nonpsychotic, eight responded completely.[129] Of the three drugs, Murphy considered aminoglutethimide the most promising and deplored the fact that it had been taken off the market (in 2004). She told the authors, in a personal communication in 2007, "I have one obsessive/compulsive patient who responded beautifully to aminoglutethimide and fluoxetine for about seven years, and has done poorly ever since AG became unavailable." She added, "Mifepristone is my least favorite antiglucocorticoid drug."[130]

Simultaneously with the kindling of Murphy's interest, other groups became curious about mifepristone's impact on the endocrine system, and, ultimately, on psychiatric illness. Their curiosity was not immediately related to drug development. In 1984, Xavier Bertagna and collaborators at several Paris hospitals, and Rolf Gaillard in the Division of Endocrinology of the University Hospital in Lausanne, Switzerland, in separate research, noted that mifepristone inhibited glucocorticoid action in humans.[131] Philip Gold, leader of the neuroendocrine branch at NIMH, followed these developments with interest and in 1989 reported the results of mifepristone in depressed patients compared to healthy volunteers. In controls there was some HPA activation: both ACTH and cortisol rose. But in depression the rise was much greater: Something about mifepristone altered the endocrine platform on which depression rests. "The capacity of depressed patients to generate robust ACTH responses to a glucocorticoid receptor antagonist suggests an alteration in the overall set point for cortisol secretion . . . as an explanation for hypercortisolism in major depression," Gold and collaborators concluded.[132]

Duke University, too, was a powerhouse of neuroendocrine research under the chairmanship of Bernard Carroll and the active collaboration of Charles Nemeroff and K. Ranga Rama Krishnan. The group looked at the effects of mifepristone in depression: Was increased cortisol a result of brain activation? They found, as Gaillard had originally suggested, that administration of mifepristone increased HPA activity: "The finding of an increase in plasma corticotropin [ACTH] and cortisol concentration after the administration of RU-486 [mifepristone] suggests that there is a suprahypophyseal drive of the hypothalamo pituitary adrenal axis in depression."[133] Again, the finding was basic neuroscience and not related to drug development (although the Duke researchers did envision a trial of mifepristone in mania, which apparently did not take place[134]). But it shows that many fast-lane research groups had picked up on the importance of mifepristone.

And as a therapeutic agent?

The scene shifts back to the Schatzberg group at McLean Hospital, originally occupied with endocrine treatments of psychotic depression. In 1991, Schatzberg moved to California as the chair of psychiatry at Stanford University; Rothschild in the meantime made his way to Worcester, Massachusetts, as professor of psychiatry at the University of Massachusetts Medical Center. Yet they remained research collaborators.

In 1998, Schatzberg helped found a private company called Corcept Therapeutics, Inc., in Menlo Park, California, with Joseph Belanoff, who had been a psychiatry resident at Stanford and who had a background in business, as the chief executive officer. (One account has Belanoff as the leading figure in founding Corcept.[135]) Belanoff and Schatzberg had a common interest in the treatment of psychotic depression; they had studied olanzapine (Lilly's antipsychotic Zyprexa) in the condition.[136] Corcept was founded around a single drug: the development of mifepristone, trade-named Corlux, for psychotic depression, later, for the "psychosis" of psychotic depression. (Rothschild later said that he had never been associated with Corcept and had merely consulted for them briefly.[137])

Corcept's expectations of mifepristone were high. Schatzberg said in 2001, "We view this as potentially ECT in a bottle."[138] The company embarked upon a series of trials. A single case of a psychotic Cushing's patient in 2001 was a spectacular success;[139] a randomly controlled trial of five patients with psychotic depression at Stanford University in that same year showed promise.[140] In October of 2001, the investigators assayed an article in the *American Journal of Psychiatry* on the distinctive cognitive profile and higher cortisol level of patients with psychotic depression.[141] After an encouraging open-label trial with mifepristone published in 2002, the company decided to sponsor a series of potentially pivotal trials for FDA licensing.[142] In 2003, Schatzberg forecast this upcoming activity in the *Journal of Clinical Psychiatry*. After discussing the disadvantages of the other treatments, he offered, "Mifepristone is a potent GR [glucocorticoid receptor] antagonist that has shown potential for rapidly reversing psychotic symptoms in delusional depression."[143]

At this writing, the larger randomly controlled trials (RCTs) have been disappointing. An RCT in 2004 involving 221 patients with psychotic depression at twenty-nine sites in the United States did not detect a difference between mifepristone and placebo in depression, although mifepristone did seem to have some effect on psychosis. The authors were dismayed by the high placebo response in a disease in which placebo responses are virtually nonexistent.[144] (A pointed note from Bernard Carroll and Robert Rubin debunked the results of this 2004 trial and Corcept's other early trials: "No study has demonstrated clinical utility for mifepristone in treating psychotic depression," they said.[145])

Another trial in 2006 in thirty seven patients recruited through the in- and outpatient services at Stanford was similarly unable to detect a difference in depression between mifepristone and placebo, although psychosis was moderately ameliorated.[146]

Given that the investigators began their careers in endocrine psychiatry with the dexamethasone test, it is curious that they did not make participation in these trials conditional upon a positive DST. Endocrine psychiatrist Uriel Halbreich remarked flatly, "The Corcept trials have all failed because they didn't control for cortisol hypersecretion."[147]

There might, however, be a genuine use for mifepristone in psychiatry after all. In 2007, a team of pharmacologists at the National Institute of Mental Health and Neurosciences in Bangalore, India, established that administering mifepristone before a convulsive treatment might attenuate the memory loss that may accompany ECT. This was a controlled trial on rats, the purpose of which was to demonstrate that "glucocorticoid mechanisms may contribute to ECT-induced retrograde amnesia."[148]

There the mifepristone story lies: a steroidal treatment of psychotic depression once thought equivalent to "ECT in a bottle." Future positive results might redeem the concept of treating brain illness via the endocrine system. Future negative results in the short term would discourage the hypothesis that psychotic depression is related to hypercortisolemia, an unhappy result for suffering patients, because cortisol does play a role in the illness.[149] In the long term, more failed trials might further diminish the flagging faith of psychiatry in the whole endocrine approach to diseases of the mind and brain.

8

The Fall of Endocrine Psychiatry

In science, time is supposed to bring us closer to knowledge. The burst of neuroendocrine research in the middle of the twentieth century should have hastened the solution of the riddle of melancholia. Instead, the opposite happened. Psychiatry lost interest in endocrine approaches. Though melancholia as a diagnosis became increasingly popular, the endocrine tide itself ebbed. This is really a rise-and-fall story. We saw endocrine theories and treatments rising from the mid-nineteenth century, as Brown-Séquard performed adrenalectomies and injected himself with animal testicular extract. We witnessed the apex of endocrine approaches in the search for biological markers that began with the dexamethasone suppression test and in the excitement surrounding the hypothalamic hormones in the 1970s and 1980s. And then the air went out of it. Neuroendocrine approaches did flourish in the new century, but among endocrinologists, not psychiatrists. The psychiatric gaze diverted elsewhere, in a discipline known for its chronically short attention span.

In 2008 one of us (Shorter) was at a psychiatric conference in Utrecht, a small town in the Netherlands. A senior Dutch psychiatrist asked me what I was working on, and I responded, "the history of the dexamethasone test. Do you use it?"

"Oh," responded my interlocutor, "That was discredited many years ago."

My heart sank. A useful diagnostic tool in psychiatry, an important biological marker in a discipline largely without a biology of psychiatric illness, seemed truly dead. Let's put on our seven-league boots and stride backward thirty years.

The year is 1980. FDA's Psychopharmacologic Drugs Advisory Committee is discussing the draft FDA guidelines on trials for antidepressant and anxiolytic drugs. Barney Carroll is a member of the advisory committee:

> By the time these guidelines are revised, which might be two to three years, I think there will be a group of laboratory diagnostic measures accepted certainly by the APA. And some mention of the appearance of diagnostic laboratory tests I think would be in order in these guidelines.
>
> .... For these guidelines ... special attention might be given to the distinction between melancholic and non-endogenous depressions in view of evidence that specific drug responses occur only in the first group.[1]

It is remarkable how history went in exactly the opposite direction from that which Carroll forecast: Psychiatry rejected laboratory tests and failed to observe the distinction between melancholia and non-melancholia to which he had called attention. Instead, "major depression" dominated the visual field. The DST and other biological markers sank from sight, for the Dutch psychiatrist in Utrecht and for many, many others.

In 2007, Steven E. Hyman, director of NIMH from 1996 to 2001, said, "Laboratory tests for the major common psychiatric disorders have not yet materialized."[2] He was not alone in this dubiety. In 1996, Herman Van Praag, former chair of psychiatry at Albert Einstein College of Medicine, told David Healy in an interview, "It is fair to say, that so far in spite of 35 years, 40 years of intensive biological research, there is no single biological variable with any diagnostic significance."[3] The burden of endocrine psychiatry is that these views are wrong.

Yet they are widely believed, and the result is that endocrine approaches have slid from the radar of today's psychiatry. A harbinger was Fred Goodwin and Kay Redfield Jamison's massive opus, *Manic-Depressive Illness*, in 1990. Goodwin was by now a senior administrator in the federal mental-health establishment; Jamison was a member of the department of psychiatry of Johns Hopkins University. Their coolness toward neuroendocrine approaches was palpable. Yes, they conceded, there had been many interesting findings about the neuroendocrinology of "depression," yet few studies elucidated differences between unipolar and bipolar illness, their main interest. Rather than focusing on differences between melancholia and non-melancholia within depression, the authors downplayed the entire endocrine enterprise by conflagrating a straw man: "It would be naïve to assume that one pathophysiological chain underlies all bipolar illness,"[4] as though anyone had made such a claim about endocrine psychiatry (although plenty had about the biogenic amine neurotransmitters).

The ACNP is a leading organization of research into the subject; its periodic volumes draw together the literature, offering a weathervane of the field's future. Endocrine themes dropped from a respectable representation in the 1970s and 1980s to virtually zero in the most recent volume in 2002 ("most recent" at the time of the publication of this book): the 2002 volume did not even have "neuroendocrine" in the index.[5]

What happened? Why has endocrine psychiatry virtually vanished from the consciousness of psychiatrists? One factor is the failure of endocrine approaches to produce new and effective drugs. When nothing of a therapeutic nature came out of the study of the adrenal steroids and the peptides—with the questionable exception of mifepristone—the profession threw its hands in the air and pronounced endocrine neurobiology of little interest as it yielded no practical results. This is tantamount to pronouncing the study of nutrition worthless because it has produced no magical weight-loss pill. As Art Prange reflected in 2007 about the failure of peptide research to pay off commercially: "There was really a very rich twenty years or so, the final ones of my career, I am happy to say. But owing partly to bad luck, partly to the wrong-headedness of Big Pharma, and partly to the nature of things, peptides and their congeners didn't pan out as treatments."[6]

In the absence of pharmaceutical treatments and big companies to promote them, the attention of the field shifted elsewhere: to genetics and neurotransmitters. "The genetic revolution has swept everything before it," said Paul McHugh, former head of psychiatry at Johns Hopkins University, in 2007. "I can't persuade people to do DSTs. I do them, but I can't get anyone else to do them."[7]

David Rubinow, chair of psychiatry at the UNC, agreed that it was the field's infatuation with genetics that had caused it to turn away from more hands-on approaches: "Everybody's interested in genetics, and everybody thinks that genetics is going to be the bio-marker Rosetta stone, that somehow we're going to be able to

genotype people, and then we're going to be able to tell their future."
Rubinow said that "very little of the variance for a disorder is going to
be in the structure of the genes."

Max Fink asked Rubinow about the study of cortisol: "It just died?"

Rubinow answered, "Yes. It did. And some of the stuff wasn't even
published and died, and it shouldn't have died. I still think that it's
amazingly interesting."[8]

But the number of people who found, as Rubinow did, the study of
cortisol "amazingly interesting" became ever fewer. Marvin Stein,
former head of psychiatry at Mount Sinai Hospital in New York, said,
"I think the field has moved into 'molecular biology' . . . with its heavy
emphasis on genetic markers, on what are the underlying molecular
faults in the brain. This department here [he gestured around him],
I don't know what the hell they're talking about. You pick up a
journal—I was at a dinner the other night with [he mentioned the
name of a former chair of psychiatry at the downstate campus]. I said
to him, 'Are you in the department of psychiatry?' and he said, 'How can
I be in the department of psychiatry? I don't know what they're doing.'"[9]

Are these voices merely the bleating holdovers of an old regime, or
are they lamenting the loss of something important in the rush to
genetics? One recalls that at the very beginning of the story, endocrine
psychiatry was associated with a whole-body approach to illness,
studying psychiatric disease not just in unconscious conflict or neurotransmitters, but in the very integuments of the body itself. That was
what Kurt Schneider envisioned in 1920 with his distinction between
reactive depression and vital depression. The latter was an affair of the
entire body, weighting down things, dragging them down, submerging
thought and mood in a sea of weariness and pain. These whole-body
perspectives are certainly no longer fashionable. Paul McHugh says,
"They don't like to look at the physiology of the organism in the midst of
a disease any more."[10]

Thus, the whole endocrine project has trickled away. Said a clinician in Scottsdale, Arizona, "One of the psychopharmacologists with
whom I work most closely and highly respect used to do TRH stimulation tests on each new patient. As I recall, the factory where they made
the TRH product burned down and the TRH hormone bolus was no
longer available."[11] And that was the end of it.

We do not mean to say that interest in melancholia has been lost
along with the slide of the endocrines. Gordon Parker and his associates
at the Black Dog Institute in Sydney, Australia, led the revival in 1996

with a comprehensive volume focusing on motor and mood symptoms of melancholia (giving the DST the back of their hand, however).[12] In 2006, Michael Alan Taylor at the University of Michigan and Max Fink wrote a historical, clinical, and biological overview of melancholia—featuring a more positive assessment of the DST—that envisioned reinserting melancholia in the official disease classification as a separate illness and using measures of cortisol abnormality as a verifier of the diagnosis (see the next chapter).[13] In 2006 as well, a conference was held in Copenhagen under the auspices of Tom Bolwig, professor of psychiatry at the University of Copenhagen, on the assessment of melancholia "beyond DSM, beyond neurotransmitters." There was great interest in the conference and its proceedings.[14] Thus melancholia, the target for which the DST is the arrow, has not evaporated at all. Quite the contrary.

Yet endocrine psychiatry languishes.

Endocrine approaches to severe depressive illness no longer register in the attention of clinicians. In February of 2006, the authors were talking with Walter Brown, a longtime biological psychiatrist at Brown University. Max Fink had a story for Dr. Brown:

> At Stony Brook [where Fink teaches] one of the attendings admitted a depressed woman, and offered her medication treatment. And on a Friday the family said they wanted to take her home. When she was admitted she was suicidal and on one-to-one observation. And after 48 hours she was on Q-15s [observation every 15 minutes]. And on Friday, the family thinks she's better, and they ask for permission for a home visit. The attending, the resident, the social worker, and the nurse meet at three o'clock in the afternoon.
>
> They say, "OK, she can have a pass, with the family." When she went out, she committed suicide.

Fink asked Brown, might there have been a role for the DST here? Brown said, "Oh, yes. This suicide thing keeps coming up. The DST is a predictor of suicide. That clearly is a clinical use for it."[15]

The desert landscape of present-day psychiatry is littered with unstable and unreliable diagnoses, a plethora of poorly effective "me, too" medications, treatment algorithms that are not evidence-based but influenced by industry marketing, unproven "therapies" in variants of psychotherapy and brain stimulation. The promises of oases of relief from the scions of neuroscience and genetics are yet to be fulfilled. It is reasonable to reexamine the well of neuroendocrinology that was passed over in ignorance and error. It is a science that offers ways to a more reliable classification of disorders, to verifying tests for diagnoses, and to guides to different treatments beyond the tweaking of neurotransmitters that excites the pharmaceutical industry and the research establishment today.

It's time to take a second look.

9

Afterword

Max Fink

How did the rise and fall in interest in endocrines affect clinicians such as myself treating the severely psychiatric ill?

As I began training, psychiatric diagnosis was descriptive, since the pathology of mental disorders was largely unknown outside the impact of infections, seizure disorders, and brain lesions. Effective treatments for the psychiatric ill were few; most treatments decreased the severity of symptoms to make living more bearable. Prescription was easy. For the non-destructive, cooperative, intelligent, and especially attractive patient, psychotherapy was advocated. For the acutely ill and severely depressed patient, especially those needing protective care, ECT was the easy choice. For the severely compromised psychotic and manic patient, insulin coma or leucotomy was offered. Bromides, barbiturates, and chloral were widely prescribed.

The explosive introduction of psychoactive drugs in the 1950s sparked the question—for whom was each agent useful? What condition called for which new agent? Within the five-year period beginning in 1953, reserpine, chlorpromazine, meprobamate, imipramine, and lysergic acid were new agents investigated at Hillside Hospital, a two-hundred-bed voluntary psychiatric hospital in Queens, New York. After training in neurology and psychiatry, I had come to the hospital in 1952 for additional experience in psychodynamic psychotherapy, the flag that the hospital flew. Insulin coma (ICT), convulsive therapy (ECT), group psychotherapy, and art therapies were also offered. I was quickly attracted to the ECT and ICT service, and in 1954 I established the hospital's EEG laboratory. NIMH funding allowed me to develop a broad research program to monitor patient treatments.[1,2] It was at Hillside that I first encountered melancholia, although at the time we were not, for the most part, calling it that.

A five-year follow-up of 317 patients admitted to the hospital in 1950 reported the diagnoses, treatments prescribed, and clinical outcomes. Psychotherapy was the mainstay treatment for 51%, insulin coma for 15%, and ECT for 34% of the patients. Psychoneurosis (37%), manic-depressive illness (17%), involutional melancholia (16%), and schizophrenia (30%) were the principal diagnoses. The average durations of stay were longest for psychoneurotic patients (7.6 months) and schizophrenia (5.7 months) and shortest for the depressive conditions (3.9 months). Those treated with ECT were discharged after an average of 5 months, with psychotherapy after 6 months and ICT after 6.5 months.[3]

We lacked identifying labels and dosing guidelines for the new agents. When the first patients were treated with chlorpromazine, we quickly noted the reductions in agitation, excitement, and delusions. Chlorpromazine dosing began at 50 mg and increased to 1200 mg/day. At this dose we effectively reduced psychosis and motor excitement in 80% of our patients within four weeks. Rigidity, posturing, and tremors marked the upper limit of dosing. We settled on procyclidine (Kemadrin) as an effective prophylactic for motor rigidity.

Nurses eagerly recommended patients for the treatment, encouraging our studies. We asked: Could chlorpromazine replace ICT, a treatment that was highly risky, with seizures, prolonged coma, and death as persistent threats? Patients referred for ICT were randomly assigned to either fifty comas or three months of daily chlorpromazine dosing. After experience with sixty patients, we reported equivalent efficacy in behavior ratings, discharge rates, and in the incidence and severity of complications. Seizures were induced in 15% of the ICT and 9% of the chlorpromazine treatment groups. Prolonged coma occurred in 10% of the ICT group. Chlorpromazine was clearly a safer treatment, easier to administer, at much less cost, and with similar outcomes to ICT; we concluded that "neither treatment altered the basic schizophrenic process, nor is there any evidence that there is a greater specificity of either form of therapy for schizophrenic illnesses."[4] Our enthusiasm for ICT ended, and the Hillside Hospital Medical Board closed the facility in 1959.[5]

We lacked criteria for the prescription of chlorpromazine and imipramine. Considering their different EEG effects, we designed a random-assignment study of chlorpromazine, imipramine, or placebo for patients referred for medication regardless of their clinical diagnosis.[6] Dosing was by fixed schedules of weekly increments up to 1200 mg/day for chlorpromazine and 300 mg/day for imipramine for a six-week treatment course. Newly developed symptom rating scales for various behaviors assessed outcomes. In our sample of 150 patients, we confirmed the antipsychotic benefit of chlorpromazine and the antidepressant benefit of imipramine. We reported an antidepressant benefit for chlorpromazine, a novel finding, which later was clarified as particularly effective in those with psychotic depression.[7] Phobias in adolescents were relieved by imipramine, a new use.[8] As psychotic adolescents became more aggressive with imipramine, we cautioned its use in this population.[9] Acute discontinuation of imipramine elicited a "flu-like" withdrawal reaction of dysphoria, aches and pains, anorexia, and lassitude, a demonstration of the development of tolerance to imipramine use.[10]

The differential efficacies indicated that it was possible to verify a presumptive diagnosis by the treatment response. In terms of pharmacotherapy, manic-depressive illness, most of which would qualify as melancholia, responded to imipramine. This method was later used by Richard Abrams and Michael Taylor[11,12,13,14] and by Donald Klein[15] in their clinical studies. Decades later, Taylor and I used treatment response to validate our arguments for the independent classification of catatonia[16,17] and of melancholia.[18,19,20]

Neuroendocrine Exploration

Although we paid attention to thyroid measures in clinical assessments of our patients, especially in patients with mental dullness and occasionally among the excited, it was the report on hypercortisolemia in melancholic depression that aroused our interest. We had been alerted to neuroendocrine abnormalities in psychiatric disorders at the 1975 meeting of the American Psychopathological Association,[21] but it was the publications by Carroll, Curtis, and Mendels[22] and Carroll's studies in Melbourne[23] that stimulated my interest. As an attending psychiatrist on an acute psychosis unit of the Northport Veterans Hospital responsible for the ECT service, I asked a research fellow Yiannis Papakostas to verify the merits of the DST. We asked the clinical laboratory to carry out the blood serum analyses following Carroll's methods, and for the next year, we applied the DST to as many patients—depressed, psychotic, and manic—from whom we could obtain voluntary consent. We excluded those with overt substance abuse, seizures, head injuries, and neurological disorders. We also examined the TSH response to injected TRH.[24] For each test, blood serum was examined on admission and before and after courses of ECT and psychotropic medications.[25]

Elevated serum cortisol and the failure to suppress with dexamethasone were recorded in ten of sixteen depressed patients referred for ECT. After treatment, the DST normalized in six. Of these, two relapsed and four remained well on follow-up. Of the four whose test remained abnormal, all had unfavorable outcomes. Years later I realized that using a fixed dosing schedule for unilateral electrode placement had offered inefficient treatments.[26]

Our findings with the TSH response to TRH were less robust. The test results did not change with effective treatment, suggesting that this measure was not as sensitive as the DST to the state of melancholia.

The Riddle of ECT

The intimate relationships among cortisol measures and illness, remission, and relapse compelled their consideration in the riddle of the ECT mechanism. How could inducing seizures impact emotional life? Early in my career, I had reported that persistent changes in EEG measures were necessary, but not sufficient, for the treatment's benefits in behavior. A decade later, the relationship between indirect measures of acetylcholine excited interest, but no function of acetylcholine could be related to the effects on mood, motor function, or thought. But when the focus shifted to the endocrine system and its intimate relationships to behavior, we saw a glimmer of an explanation. It was slow in coming.

A 1972 NIMH conference on the ECT mechanism examined the effects of seizures on brain neurotransmitters, electrophysiology, and memory, the functions that were then thought important for the therapeutic chain.[27] The changes in electrophysiology and memory accompanying seizures were considered side-effects. The rise in brain epinephrine, norepinephrine, acetylcholine, and corticoid levels with each seizure were deemed coincidental, not central, findings. Increased cerebrovascular permeability, cerebral hypoxia, and changes in mineral and water metabolism were targeted as consequences of the seizures that may contribute to the outcome. The most optimistic suggestions came from the clinical studies of vegetative functions that are often awry in psychiatric disorders—weight, appetite, sleep, digestion, libido, and menstruation. Abnormalities in these functions were associated with a good response to ECT, improved rapidly with successful treatment, and were related to the amount of EEG seizure activity. No participant discussed the role of the body's hormone systems.

These systems were first considered at the second NIMH conference on ECT in New Orleans in 1978.[28] Jan-Otto Ottosson described how lidocaine blocked the EEG effects of seizures and also reduced the behavioral effect. The symmetry of the brain seizure activity directed attention to the diencephalon.[29] Increasing the EEG effects by administering barbiturates enhanced the antidepressant effect.[30] Subconvulsive currents and asymmetrical brain stimulation (as in unilateral ECT) failed to elicit EEG changes necessary for behavioral improvement. The functions of the brain stem became the target of interest in convulsive therapy.[31] The role of the master neuroendocrine glands compelled attention to the endocrines to explain the effects of ECT.[32]

The failure of imipramine to relieve psychotic depression encouraged this formulation. When hospitalized depressed patients were treated with imipramine at doses monitored by serum levels for adequacy, some failed to respond but did recover with ECT. The imipramine non-responders were the psychotic depressed.[33] An earlier Italian study had also reported that psychotic depressed patients were imipramine non-responders.[34] These observations were quickly confirmed, and we became aware that psychotic depression differed from non-psychotic depression in more ways than severity.[35] Almost all psychotic depressed patients exhibited hypercortisolemia and lacked suppression with dexamethasone, while in the non-psychotic depressed the test results were often within normal limits.[36]

Supporting evidence for the role of neuroendocrines appeared sporadically, a commentary on the stepchild status to which ECT research has been relegated. Interest in the role of neurotransmitters in psychoactive agents dominated research as the effects of antidepressant drugs were thought to reside in the enhancement of the brain's monoaminergic activity.[37]

To measure the impact of seizures on hypothalamic function, I obtained cerebrospinal fluid from patients before and after six ECT. With successful treatment in nine depressed patients, the CSF levels of somatostatin increased, and both CRF and beta-endorphin decreased.[38] (Somatostatin is low in depressed patients.) Case reports note the changes in an abnormal DST and resolution of depression with one ECT.[39]

A decade later, the neuroendocrine hypothesis was criticized as too non-specific to be testable, a complaint that reflected the shift in interest from neuroendocrine physiology to brain receptor chemistry.[40] But no alternative explanation for ECT has surfaced. The efficacy of ECT for patients unresponsive to psychoactive medications expanded its use, but interest in its mechanism faded. Sadly, the research interest in ECT continued chiefly on technical issues to reduce side-effects, leaving the practice almost unchanged from three decades ago.[41]

Clinical Experience in the 1980s and 1990s

In 1980, I assumed responsibility for the ECT service of a thirty-bed inpatient adult unit at University Hospital at Stony Brook, New York. I brought the DST methodology from the VA Hospital studies. From time to time, I used the DST to support decisions as to the end of the treatment course and to justify renewed treatments with the early signs of relapse. I found the DST useful in deciding individual treatment protocols.

By the early 1990s, however, the complexities of reimbursement forced the Department to pay for these tests from non-clinical research funds. Suddenly, requesting the DST became a research, not a clinical, decision. The political decisions by the APA and NIMH committees described earlier in this volume had borne bitter fruit. Later in the decade the NIMH extramural program supported multicenter colla-borative studies of continuation treatments after ECT and variations in electrode placement in a study program known as CORE.[42] Support to examine cortisol was requested in the two studies, but funding for these tests was refused, forcing the clinical studies to proceed without a biological measure.[43] Interest in the DST had collapsed.

Shift to Psychopathology

After retiring from the Stony Brook clinical services, I wrote a new ECT text, intended for patients and their families.[44] I reassessed the literature on the mechanism of ECT, finding that the alternative explanations had garnered little support, while the neuroendocrine view was the most viable.[45] Jointly with Jan-Otto Ottosson of Sweden, we debated the ethics of ECT.[46]

While in charge of the ECT service at Stony Brook University Hospital in 1987, I was asked to examine a young woman with lupus erythematosus in a malignant manic and catatonic state requiring sedation, restraints, and parenteral feeding. ECT was offered, accepted by her family, and the syndrome resolved.[47] This experience stimulated interest in catatonia.[48]

The parallel between melancholia and catatonia is quite interesting. Both once stood prominently center-stage in psychiatric classification; both then fell into desuetude as the attention of the field glanced elsewhere; both are experiencing a revival today. Melancholia, the subject of the present volume, has a powerful neuroendocrine component. There is some evidence that catatonia may as well. This parallel thus leads me to beg the reader's indulgence for a few more lines about catatonia, which was described in 1874 by the German psychopathologist Karl Kahlbaum. Within a few years the syndrome was recognized in from 8 percent to 38 percent of large samples of hospitalized patients. It then seemed to disappear, and observers assumed that the introduction of antipsychotic drugs successfully eliminated catatonia from the clinic.[49] In the 1970s, however, catatonia was increasingly reported, first in manic and depressed patients and then in those with the neurotoxic syndrome labeled "neuroleptic malignant syndrome." Catatonia had not disappeared but was no longer recognized, mainly because clinical emphasis had shifted from the severely hospitalized psychiatric ill to anxious and depressed outpatient populations. Office practice did not encourage systemic medical examination or the testing that is essential for the recognition of catatonia.[50]

To assess the incidence of catatonia on an inpatient academic service, we developed a rating scale to identify and quantify its severity. A year's survey of 215 inpatient admissions to our university hospital found 9 percent to exhibit catatonia.[51] Almost all the patients met criteria for affective illness (more often mania than depression) or a toxic response (most often to neuroleptic drugs but also in systemic illnesses). Fewer than 10 percent met criteria for schizophrenia, supporting the earlier studies that populations exhibiting catatonia more often met criteria for affective illness than for schizophrenia.[52] The classification of catatonia only as a type of schizophrenia in *DSM-III* had erred.

Joining with Michael Taylor, one of the clinicians in the 1970s who had described catatonia more often in manic patients, we urged the *DSM-IV* Commission of the APA to consider catatonia as an independent syndrome, much like delirium and dementia.[53] The Commission did not agree but did add a class of "catatonia secondary to a medical illness" and as a modifier of affective illnesses.[54] These adjustments of the classification did not recognize the independent nature of catatonia. In 2003 we again recommended an independent class for catatonia, "a home of its own" in the next iteration of the psychiatric classification[55] and repeated that recommendation in 2006.[56]

Catatonia, like melancholia, is eminently identifiable and treatable.[57] In 1930, high doses of parenteral amobarbital were described as immediately relieving the mutism, posturing, and negativism of catatonia. [58] A few years later, the rapid efficacy of convulsive therapy was reported.[59] In time, amobarbital was replaced by lorazepam and diazepam. In our studies, an intravenous bolus of lorazepam transiently relieved catatonia in more than 80 percent of our subjects, and we suggested that such a challenge be considered a verifying test of the syndrome. High doses of oral lorazepam successfully sustained relief, although a few patients still required ECT.[60] With this experience, it was possible to identify catatonia as a syndrome by its motor signs, verify the diagnosis by a lorazepam challenge test, and successfully treat the syndrome by benzodiazepines—and, when those failed, with ECT. The responsiveness of both catatonia and melancholia to convulsive therapy is quite interesting and suggestive of some common underlying mechanism. The riddle of melancholia, in other words, is entwined with the riddle of catatonia.

Catatonia is a definable syndrome with diverse faces.[61] Although the acute neuroleptic malignant syndrome was initially thought to be a dopaminergic imbalance in response to neuroleptics, the similarities of the syndrome to malignant catatonia and the successful response to benzodiazepines and ECT suggest that the underlying cause is the catatonic process.[62] The mutism, negativism, posturing, staring, and repetitive self-injurious behavior of adolescents with mental retardation and autism-spectrum disorders are increasingly recognized as signs of catatonia; ECT has relieved these patients of their self-destructive behavior and materially improved their quality of life. [63] Catatonia is also increasingly recognized among patients with delirium, admitted either to the psychiatric services in delirious mania or on the medical and surgical services where they require intensive treatment.[64]

We know little about the neuroendocrine features of catatonia. In malignant catatonia, fever, occasionally to fatal levels; hypertension; tachycardia; and tachypnea are evidence that the autonomic system is disorganized. Patients are often in stupor. A few case reports assess cortisol levels, but we lack systematic studies.[70] Finding the neuroendocrine basis for catatonia is a challenge that commands attention.

Melancholia

While celebrating the publication of *Catatonia*, Taylor and I mused whether another psychiatric syndrome might lend itself to the same intensive review. Melancholia was such a syndrome, and the alliteration of "catatonia" and "melancholia" resonated. We divided the topic chapters, and I accepted the challenges of describing the syndrome's history and neuroendocrine studies.[66]

Hypercortisolemia was recognized as a sign in pituitary adenoma, still a clinically useful test. The subsequent finding of high and even higher levels of cortisol in severely depressed patients and the development of the DST as a marker of melancholic depression, its severity, and remission and relapse quickly excited the research community.[67] The initial studies were quickly verified, and hypercortisolemia was seen as a marker of the active phase of the melancholia syndrome. All this is described extensively in the previous chapters. Although hypercortisolemia had been discarded in the clinic, our review of the experience impressed us as verifying a specific psychiatric syndrome. We focused attention on the classical syndrome that had been recognized in centuries of medical writing. That melancholia is eminently treatable when separated from non-melancholic depressions—meaning depressions without cortisol abnormality as their root—is an incidental but very valuable benefit.

We recognized that the DST methodology has limitations, yet we concluded that a positive test verifies the diagnosis of melancholia much as the EEG verifies a seizure disorder or the ECG a cardiac event.[73] As we saw in previous chapters, ongoing studies to optimize the DST assess dexamethasone dosage and metabolism. Augmentation by CRF or dextroamphetamine, biochemical measurements, and time of sampling: all hold the promise of improving the usefulness of abnormal cortisol metabolism in the identification of melancholia.

The failure to separate melancholia and non-melancholic depressions impairs clinical treatment trials. The recent government-sponsored multi-site collaborative study known as STAR*D failed to identify an antidepressant benefit for the new SSRI agents; indeed, the agents elicited improvement rates similar to that of placebo.[69] The heterogeneity of the populations was a significant factor in the failure of the studies.

The studies of mifepristone, an antiglucocorticoid and antiprogestogen agent that blocks the gluticocorticoid receptor as a treatment for psychotic depression, have been similarly flawed. Mifepristone was examined for the benefit that might accrue when cortisol action was blocked. If this mechanism is anticipated, it would be logical to examine patients with melancholia, with specific evidence of hypercortisolemia. But this was not done in the multicenter clinical trials that failed to show a benefit compared to that enjoyed by the placebo.[70]

Clinically useful relationships have been found for neuroendocrine measures and psychiatric treatments. These tests hold promise for improving clinical practice and treatment assessments. But studies that sought to apply the endocrine tests as measures of the *DSM*'s fanciful and capricious "disorders" were interpreted as a failure of the test, not the failure to assure diagnostic homogeneity in applying the diagnostic criteria. Neuroendocrine tests were discarded, to the unpardonable disadvantage of clinicians in their treatment choices and in their care of the psychiatric ill.

L'envoi

Nature yields new findings in medical science grudgingly, and to discard a finding because it does not serve a wished-for purpose, to discard hypercortisolemia in melancholia because it fails the test of identifying the fantasized "major depression" and "bipolar disorder" of the *DSM-III* commissioners, is wasteful and unforgivable. Endocrine findings direct our attention to the body's hormonal systems as sources of the illnesses that populate the psychiatric clinics, hospitals, and asylums. Endocrine measures are directly applicable within the medical model of diagnosis. They constitute sophisticated metrics of a specific syndrome of melancholia, a mood disorder that is now submerged under the rubrics of major depression and bipolar disorder. Identifying melancholia in a patient promises the relief of remission, something that is unknown for the non-melancholic depressive disorders. Assessing hormone dysregulation in the mood disorders warrants renewed attention, first to improve the definition of melancholia, then to improve the measurements, and finally as a model for similar aberrances for other conditions in the psychiatric clinic.

"Treatment response," one element of the medical model of diagnosis proposed by Robins and Guze, warrants greater attention in identifying populations for clinical classification purposes.[71] Its rejection as a measure by the *DSM* classification system is reckless and unjustified.

While the present trend in psychiatric classification favors "splitters"—each iteration of the *DSM* classification has increased the number of "disorders"[72]—the application of verification tests and treatment responses favors "lumping" disorders together. This benefit is well demonstrated by the variety of disorders that meet our criteria for catatonia and encourage effective treatments. A similar variety of disorders meets criteria for melancholia, to the benefit of patients who can now be treated effectively.

The split of the nineteenth-century manic-depressive illness into two different kinds of depression—unipolar and bipolar—denies the clinical reality that melancholic depression is commonly associated with manic features, and a mixed manic-depressive syndrome is widely acknowledged. Identifying melancholia as a mood disorder with motor and vegetative features, marked by cortisol abnormality and validated by treatment response to tricyclic antidepressants and to ECT, usefully separates melancholic and non-melancholic mood disorders.

The evidence that the neuroendocrine system is affected in psychiatric disorders, and that ECT influences the neuroendocrine system, is compelling. The neuroendocrine hypothesis underlying mood disorders and our understanding of the efficacy of convulsive therapy deserves greater attention. Indeed, accepting the response to convulsive therapy as evidence of a common pathophysiology, whether expressed as melancholia, mania, or catatonia, urges study of the neuroendocrine aspects as a key to understanding the pathophysiology of major psychiatric syndromes and clarification of the classification muddle that besets the discipline.

Notes

Abbreviations Used in Notes

AJP   *American Journal of Psychiatry*
BMJ   *British Medical Journal*
JAMA   *Journal of the American Medical Association*

Notes to Preface

1. Michael Alan Taylor and Max Fink, *Melancholia: The Diagnosis, Pathophysiology, and Treatment of Depressive Illness* (Cambridge, U.K.: Cambridge University Press, 2006), 15.
2. Edward Shorter and David Healy, *Shock Treatment: A History of Electroconvulsive Therapy in Mental Illness* (New Brunswick, N.J.: Rutgers University Press, 2007).

Notes to Chapter 1

1. Hugh B. McIntyre et al., "Computer Analyzed EEG in Amphetamine-Responsive Hyperactive Children," *Psychiatry Research*, 4 (1981): 189–197.
2. Edward Shorter and David Healy, *Shock Therapy: A History of Electroconvulsive Treatment in Mental Illness* (New Brunswick, N.J.: Rutgers University Press, 2007); Max Fink, *Electroshock: Restoring the Mind* (New York: Oxford University Press, 1999).
3. See, however, Chandak Sengoopta, *The Most Secret Quintessence of Life: Sex, Glands, and Hormones, 1850–1950* (Chicago: University of Chicago Press, 2006), a critical account of the development of the understanding of the gonadal hormones; Victor Cornelius Medvei, *A History of Endocrinology* (Lancaster, Pa.: MTP Press, 1982), which gives rather little attention to recent neuroendocrinology; and Alison Li, "Wondrous Transformations: Endocrinology after Insulin," in *Essays in Honour of*

Michael Bliss: Figuring the Social, ed. E[lspeth] A. Heaman, Alison Li, and Shelley McKellar (Toronto: University of Toronto Press, 2008), 351–377.

4. Edward Shorter, *Before Prozac: The Troubled History of Mood Disorders in Psychiatry* (New York: Oxford University Press, 2009).

5. Paula Clayton interview, by Edward Shorter and Max Fink, in Hollywood, Fla., Dec. 4, 2006.

6. Max Fink, "Editorial: Should the Dexamethasone Suppression Test Be Resurrected?" *Acta Psychiatrica Scandinavica*, 112 (2005): 245–249; quote, 248.

7. Joel Elkes, "Towards Footings in a New Science," interview, in *The Psychopharmacologists*, ed. David Healy, vol. 2 (London: Chapman and Hall, 1998), 183–213; quote, 188.

8. Karl (Károly) Schaffer, "Zur Pathogenese der Tay-Sachs'schen amaurotischen Idiotie," *Neurologisches Centralblatt*, 24 (1905): 386–393, 437–448.

9. Paul M. Plotsky, Michael J. Owens, and Charles B. Nemeroff, "Neuropeptide Alterations in Mood Disorders," in *Psychopharmacology: The Fourth Generation of Progress*, ed. Floyd E. Bloom and David J. Kupfer (New York: Raven, 1995), 971–981; quote, 974.

10. Richard P. Michael and James L. Gibbons, "Interrelationships Between the Endocrine System and Neuropsychiatry," *International Review of Neurobiology*, 5 (1963): 243–302; quote, 243–244.

11. Vincenzo Chiarugi, *On Insanity and Its Classification* (1793–1794), trans. with a foreword and introduction by George Mora (Canton, Mass.: Science History Pub, 1987), 257–258.

12. Henry Maudsley, *The Physiology and Pathology of the Mind* (New York: Appleton, 1867), v, 214–215.

13. Kurt Schneider, "Die Schichtung des emotionalen Lebens und der Aufbau der Depressionszustände," *Zeitschrift für die gesamte Neurologie und Psychiatrie*, 59 (1920): 281–286; Schneider, "Der Begriff der Reaktion in der Psychiatrie," *Zeitschrift für Neurologie*, 95 (1925): 500–505. For a brief summary of these concepts, see Edward Shorter, *Historical Dictionary of Psychiatry* (New York: Oxford University Press, 2005), 83.

14. Colleen Kelly, testimony, Neurological Devices Panel of the Medical Devices Advisory Committee, Food and Drug Administration, June 15, 2004, 17: available at http://www.fda.gov/ohrms/dockets/ac/04/minutes/4047m1.pdf (accessed Jan. 1, 2008).

15. Paul Ehrlich, "Ansprache bei Einweihung des Georg-Speyer-Hauses" (1906), in *The Collected Papers of Paul Ehrlich*, ed. F. Himmelweit et al., vol. 3 (London: Pergamon, 1960), 42–52; "Zauberkugeln," 49.

16. Joel Elkes, "Epilogue: On Specificity and Communication: Reflections on the Place of Languages in Psychopharmacology," in *The Neurotransmitter Era in Neuropsychopharmacology*, ed. Thomas A. Ban and Ronaldo Ucha Udabe (Buenos Aires: Polemos, 2006), 255–263; quote, 259.

Notes to Chapter 2

1. Philip W. Gold and David R. Rubinow, "Neuropeptide Function in Affective Illness: Corticotropin-Releasing Hormone and Somatostatin as Model Systems," in *Psychopharmacology: The Third Generation of Progress*, ed. Herbert Y. Meltzer (New York: Raven, 1987), 617–627; quote, 617.

2. Charles Bell, *Idea of a New Anatomy of the Brain* (London: Strahan, 1811); on the significance of this discovery, see Edwin Clarke and L. S. Jacyna, *Nineteenth-Century*

Origins of Neuroscientific Concepts (Berkeley: University of California Press, 1987), 119–113.

3. On reflex theory in psychiatry, see Edward Shorter, *From Paralysis to Fatigue: A History of Psychosomatic Illness in the Modern Era* (New York: Free Press, 1992), 20–68.

4. Andrew Scull, *Madhouse: A Tragic Tale of Megalomania and Modern Medicine* (New Haven, Conn.: Yale University Press, 2005).

5. Wilhelm Griesinger, *Pathologie und Therapie der psychischen Krankheiten* (Stuttgart, Germany: A Krabbe, 1845; 2nd [rev.] ed., Stuttgart: A. Krabbe, 1861), 55, 162–163.

6. John Simon, *A Physiological Essay on the Thymus Gland* (London: Renshaw, 1845), 98–99.

7. Arnold Adolph Berthold, "Transplantation der Hoden," *Archiv für Anatomie, Physiologie und wissenschaftliche Medizin*, 1849 [no vol. number]: 42–46.

8. [Thomas] Addison, "Anemia—Disease of the Supra-renal Capsules," *London Medical Gazette*, 43 (1849): 517–518.

9. Charles G. Gross, "Claude Bernard and the Constancy of the Internal Environment," *The Neuroscientist*, 4 (1998): 380–385.

10. [Charles]-É[douard] Brown-Séquard, "Recherches expérimentales sur la physiologie et la pathologie des capsules surrénales," *Comptes rendus hebdomadaires des séances de l'Académie des Sciences* [Paris], 43 (1856): 422–425, 542–546.

11. Charles-Édouard Brown-Séquard, "Des effets produits chez l'homme par des injections sous-cutanées d'un liquide retiré des testicules frais de cobaye et de chien," *Comptes rendus hebdomadaires des séances et mémoires de la Société de Biologie et de ses Filiales*, 41 (1889): 415–422; quote, 418.

12. [Charles-Édouard] Brown-Séquard, "Remarques sur les effets produits sur la femme par des injections sous-cutanées d'un liquid retiré d'ovaires d'animaux," *Archives de physiologie normale et pathologique*, 22 (1890): 456–457.

13. Hans Lisser, "The Endocrine Society: The First Forty Years (1917–1957)," *Endocrinology*, 80 (1967): 5–28; quote, 7.

14. William W. Gull, "On a Cretinoid State Supervening in Adult Life in Women," *Transactions of the Clinical Society of London*, 7 (1874): 180–185; quotes, 180–181, 185; the paper was given in 1873.

15. Antonio-Maria Bettencourt-Rodrigues and José-Antonio Serrano, "Un cas de myxoedème traité par la greffe hypodermique du corps thyroïde d'un mouton," *La Semaine médicale*, 10 (Aug. 13, 1890): 294.

16. George R. Murray, "Note on the Treatment of Myxoedema by Hypodermic Injections of an Extract of the Thyroid Gland of a Sheep," *BMJ*, 2 (Oct. 10, 1891): 796–797; quote, 797.

17. William Maddock Bayliss and Ernest Starling, "The Chemical Regulation of the Secretory Process," *Proceedings of the Royal Society of Medicine*, B 73 (1904): 310–322.

18. Ernest H. Starling, "The Croonian Lectures on the Chemical Correlation of the Functions of the Body, Lecture I," *Lancet*, 2 (Aug. 5, 1905): 339–341; quote, 340. On the founding of endocrinology in England, see John Henderson, "Ernest Starling and 'Hormones': An Historical Commentary," *Journal of Endocrinology*, 184 (2005): 5–10.

19. Henry Maudsley, *Body and Mind: An Inquiry in to Their Connection and Mutual Influence, Specifically in Reference to Mental Disorders* (London: Macmillan, 1870); quote, 85–86.

20. T[homas] S. Clouston, *Clinical Lectures on Mental Diseases*, 2nd ed. (London: Churchill, 1887; first ed., 1883), 486.

21. See Ian R. Dowbiggin, *Keeping America Sane: Psychiatry and Eugenics in the United States and Canada, 1880–1940* (Ithaca, N.Y.: Cornell University Press, 1997); Philip R. Reilly, *The Surgical Solution: A History of Involuntary Sterilization in the United States* (Baltimore, Md.: Johns Hopkins, 1991).

22. See Gunnar Broberg and Nils Roll-Hansen, *Eugenics and the Welfare State: Sterilization Policy in Denmark, Sweden, Norway, and Finland* (East Lansing: Michigan State University Press, 1996).

23. Medvei's standard history of endocrinology barely touches on Laignel-Lavastine. Yet no previous researcher succeeded in pulling the various endocrine disorders into a single system to explain mental illness as comprehensively as Laignel. See Victor Cornelius Medvei, *A History of Endocrinology* (Lancaster, Pa.: MTP Press, 1982).

24. On Laignel's life, see Jean Vinchon, "Maxime Laignel-Lavastine: Nécrologie," *Presse médicale,* 61 (Nov. 21, 1953): 1545; Ivolino de Vasconcelos, "Laignel-Lavastine, Mestra da Neurologia e da História da Medicina," *A Medicina Contemporânea,* 78 (1960): 511–516.

25. M[axime] Laignel-Lavastine, "Introduction à l'étude des rapports psychoglandulaires," *Revue de psychiatrie et de psychologie expérimentale,* 12 (1908): 373–378.

26. M[axime] Laignel-Lavastine, "Sécrétions internes et psychoses," *Presse médicale,* Aug. 1, 1908 [no vol. number]: 491.

27. M[axime] Laignel-Lavastine, "Les Troubles glandulaires dans les syndromes neuro-psychiatriques," *Tribune médicale,* [no vol. number], no. 37 (1908): 565–566.

28. M[axime] Laignel-Lavastine, "Les Troubles psychiques dans les syndromes thyroidiens," Congrès des Aliénistes et Neurologistes de France, *Rapports et comptes rendus,* 17 (1908): 204–230, see especially 211–212.

29. M[axime] Laignel-Lavastine, "Les Troubles de glandes à sécrétion interne chez les mélancoliques," *Revue de psychiatrie et de psychologie expérimentale,* 12 (1908): 429–433; quote, 429–430.

30. M[axime] Laignel-Lavastine, "Psychiatrie et sympathologie," *Annales médico-psychologiques,* 101 (1943): 115–137.

31. M[axime] Laignel-Lavastine, "Traitement médicamenteux des sympathoses et homéopathie," *Schweizer Archiv für Neurologie und Psychiatrie,* 27 (1931): 180–181.

32. W[illiam] H[enry] B[utter] Stoddart, "Physical Signs in Melancholia," *Journal of Mental Science,* 44 (1898): 247–259; quotes, 248, 252, 253.

33. Maurice Craig, head of psychiatry at Guy's Hospital, commented on Stoddart's findings in his textbook but was uninterested in them as a predictive biological test. Craig, *Psychological Medicine,* 3rd ed. (Philadelphia: Blakiston, 1917), 86. Theophile Raphael, apparently unaware of Stoddart's work, found that dementia praecox patients had the same minimal reactions to small doses of pilocarpine as normal subjects. Raphael, "Reaction in Dementia Praecox to Vagotonic and Sympathicotonic Criteria," *American Journal of Insanity,* 77 (1921): 543–544. Likewise, D. H. Funkenstein and co-workers, who proposed the "epinephrine-mecholyl" test of autonomic hypo- or hyper-reactivity as a sign of psychiatric illness, do not cite Stoddart. Daniel H. Funkenstein, Milton Greenblatt, and Harry C. Solomon, "Psychophysiological Study of Mentally Ill Patients, Part I: The Status of the Peripheral Autonomic Nervous System as Determined by the Reaction to Epinephrine and Mecholyl," *AJP,* 106 (1949): 16–28; Funkenstein, Greenblatt, Steven Root, and Solomon, "Part II: Changes in the Reactions to Epinephrine and Mecholyl After Electric Shock Treatment," AJP, 106(1949): 116–121. See also Leo Alexander, *Treatment of Mental Disorder* (Philadelphia: Saunders, 1953), 25–30.

34. Harvey Cushing, "Psychic Disturbances Associated with Disorders of the Ductless Glands," *American Journal of Insanity,* 69 (1913): 965–990; quotes, 969, 971, 975, 980, 989.

35. Emil Kraepelin and Johannes Lange, *Psychiatrie,* 9th ed. (Leipzig: Barth, 1927), vol. 2; quote, 1313.

36. G[eorges] Naudascher and E[mmanuel] Martimor, "Variations de la pression artérielle d'après certains états émotifs," *Annales médico-psychologiques*, ser. 11, vol. 2 (1921): 170–176.

37. G[eorges] Naudascher, "La Pression artérielle habituelle dans les états dépressifs," *L'Encéphale*, 18 (1923): 516–524.

38. Edward A. Strecker and Baldwin L. Keyes, "Ovarian Therapy in Involutional Melancholia," *New York Medical Journal and Medical Record*, 116 (1922): 30–34; quote, 34.

39. [Julius] Wagner-Jauregg, "Organotherapie bei Neurosen und Psychosen," *Wiener Klinische Wochenschrift*, 36 (Jan. 4, 1923): 1–4.

40. Gilbert Robin, "Du traitement de quelques psychoses et psychonévroses par l' opothérapie spermatogénique," *La Clinique*, 23 (1928): 171–172; quote, 172.

41. K[enneth] K[irkpatrick] Drury and C. Farran-Ridge, "Some Observations on the Types of Blood-Sugar Curve found in Different Forms of Insanity," *Journal of Mental Science*, 71 (1925): 8–29, quotes 21, 29.

42. L[ászló] J. Meduna, *Oneirophrenia* (Urbana: University of Illinois Press, 1950).

43. L[ászló] J. Meduna, *Carbon Dioxide Therapy* (Springfield, Ill.: Thomas, 1950).

44. K[arl] Kleist, "Autochthone Degenerationspsychosen," *Zeitschrift für die gesamte Neurologie und Psychiatrie*, 69 (1921): 1–11—see p. 7, where he cites in support of his views Georg Ewald's use of the Abderhaldensche Reaktion. Abderhalden himself, however, was later shown to be a scientific fraud. Ute Deichmann and Benno Müller-Hill, "The Fraud of Abderhalden's Enzymes," *Nature*, 393 (May 14, 1998): 109–111.

45. Kurt Schneider, "Die Schichtung des emotionalen Lebens und der Aufbau der Depressionszustände," *Zeitschrift für die gesamte Neurologie und Psychiatrie*, 59 (1920): 281–286.

46. Josef Westermann, "Ueber die vitale Depression," *Zeitschrift für die gesamte Neurologie und Psychiatrie*, 77 (1922): 391–422.

47. National Institutes of Health: NIH News, "Schizophrenia and Bipolar Disorder Share Genetic Roots," http://www.nih.gov/news/health/ju12009/nimh-01. htm, July 1, 2009 (accessed July 7, 2009).

48. Erich David, "Ueber die Pathogenese von Angstzuständen, sowie über ihre Therapie," *Psychiatrisch-Neurologische Wochenschrift*, 26 (June 12, 1926): 261–266; despite the title, the article discussed melancholia extensively. On Anermon and Gynormon, see F. Luthe et al., "Morphiumentziehungsbehandlung mit Anermon und Gynormon," *Medizinische Klinik*, 27 (July 10, 1931): 1038–1040.

49. Paul Büchler, "Affektpsychose und vegetativ-endokrine Störungen," *Archiv für Psychiatrie und Nervenkrankheiten*, 86 (1929): 654–664. He doesn't cite his 1922 publication, which apparently was in Hungarian.

50. "Suprarrenin" advertisement, *Wiener Medizinische Wochenschrift*, 63 (May 3, 1913): 1162.

51. "Antithyreoidin-Moebius" advertisement, *Wiener Medizinische Wochenschrift*, 63 (May 10, 1913): 1218. On its composition, see *Rote Liste 1939: Preisverzeichnis deutscher pharmazeutischer Spezialpräparate*, 3rd ed. (Berlin: Fachgruppe Pharmazeutische Erzeugnisse, 1939), 44.

52. "Pituglandol-Roche" advertisement, *Wiener Medizinische Wochenschrift*, 63 (June 21, 1913): 1591.

53. R[ufus] L. McQuillan, *Is the Doctor In? The Story of a Drug Detail Man's Fifty Years of Public Relations with Doctors and Druggists* (New York: Exposition, 1963), 57.

54. Michael Bliss, *Harvey Cushing: A Life in Surgery* (Toronto: University of Toronto Press, 2005), 382.

55. Harvey Cushing, "The Basophil Adenomas of the Pituitary Body and Their Clinical Manifestations (Pituitary Basophilism)," *Johns Hopkins Hospital Bulletin*, 50 (1932): 137–195, quotes 177, 192.

56. Ralph Gerard, "European Tour, Survey of Science in Relation to Neuro-Psychiatry (1934–35)," 101–102; manuscript in the Ralph W. Gerard Collection, Department of Special Collections, University of California, Irvine, box II-D.

57. Ibid., 110.

58. Ibid., 185.

59. R[olf] Gjessing, "Beiträge zur Kenntnis der Pathophysiologie des katatonen Stupors," *Archiv für Psychiatrie und Nervenkrankheiten*, 96 (1932); Mitteilungen I and II, 319–392, 393–473.

60. Gerard, "European Tour," 227.

61. Ted Morgan, *Maugham* (New York: Simon and Schuster, 1980); quote, 422. At this writing, La Clinique La Prairie still exists, dispensing "l'Extrait CLP" to a wide-flung clientele.

62. E[rich] Grafe, "Stoffwechselstörungen und innere Sekretion," in *Stoffwechselkrankheiten*, ed. G. Herxheimer (Berlin: Karger, 1926), 266–277; quote, 266.

63. Paul Schmidt, "Über Organtherapie und Insulinbehandlung bei endogenen Geistesstörungen," *Klinische Wochenschrift*, 7 (Apr. 29, 1928): 839–842.

64. Herbert Sack, "Organtherapeutische Ergebnisse bei depressiven Psychosen von Frauen," *Monatsschrift für Psychiatrie*, 83 (1932): 305–374.

65. O[tto] Wuth, "Körpergewicht. Endokrines System. Stoffwechsel," in *Handbuch der Geisteskrankheiten*, ed. Oswald Bumke, vol. 3 (Berlin: Springer, 1928), Allgemeiner Teil, part 3: Körperliche Störungen, 154–217; quote, 160. (In the somewhat confusing numbering of this long series, this volume represents part 3 of vol. 3.)

66. M[anfred] Bleuler, *Endokrinologische Psychiatrie* (Stuttgart, Germany: Thieme, 1954), quotes, 98–99.

67. Medvei, *History of Endocrinology*, 502. The wag was Herbert Ripley.

68. Herbert S. Ripley, Ephraim Shorr, and George N. Papanicolaou, "The Effect of Treatment of Depression in the Menopause with Estrogenic Hormone," *AJP*, 96 (1940): 905–911.

69. Heinz E. Lehmann, "Before They Called It Psychopharmacology," *Neuropsychopharmacology*, 8 (1993): 291–303.

Notes to Chapter 3

1. These biographical details are from Miriam Rothschild, "Tadeus Reichstein, 20 July 1897–1 Aug. 1996," *Biographical Memoirs of Fellows of the Royal Society*, 45 (Nov. 1999): 450–467, esp. 452, 455.

2. See W[ilbur] W. Swingle and J[oseph] J. Pfiffner, "Studies on the Adrenal Cortex, IV," *American Journal of Physiology*, 98 (1931): 144–152; quote, 152.

3. T[adeus] Reichstein, "Über Bestandteile der Nebennieren-Rinde (X): Zur Kenntnis des Cortico-sterons," *Helvetia Chimica Acta*, 20 (1937): 953–969. In 1938, Kendall observed that Reichstein's Substance M is "our Compound F." Harold Mason, Williard M. Hoehn, and Edward C. Kendall, "Chemical Studies of the Suprarenal Cortex: IV. Structures of Compounds C, D, E, F, and G," *Journal of Biological Chemistry*, 124 (1938): 459–474; see the table of equivalences on p. 467. At that point none of the competing groups had succeeded in synthesizing cortisol. On these events, see the Nobel Prize lectures that Kendall and Reichstein

delivered in 1950. Reichstein, "Chemistry of the Adrenal Cortex Hormones," *Nobel Lectures, Physiology or Medicine, 1942–1962* (Amsterdam: Elsevier, 1964), 291–308; Kendall, "The Development of Cortisone as a Therapeutic Agent," ibid., 270–288. For an overview of the discovery of the adrenocortocoids, see Bela Issekutz, *Die Geschichte der Arzneimittelforschung* (Budapest: Akademiai Kiado, 1971), 419–424.

4. For their first report, see W[ilbur] W. Swingle and J[oseph] J. Pfiffner, "Experiments with an Active Extract of the Suprarenal Cortex," *Anatomical Record*, 44 (1929): 225–226; see also Swingle and Pfiffner, "Studies on the Adrenal Cortex, IV: Further Observations on the Preparation and Chemical Properties of the Cortical Hormone," *American Journal of Physiology*, 98 (1931): 145–152.

5. Conrad A. Loehner, "Further Observations on the Use of Adrenal Cortex Extract in the Psychotic and Non-Psychotic Patient," *Endocrinology*, 27 (1940): 378–380.

6. Walter Sneader, *Drug Discovery: A History* (New York: Wiley, 2005), 180.

7. According to Leo Hollister, medical investigator at the Palo Alto Veterans Hospital, "In the older literature, it was commonly said that in most patients thought to have manic-depressive disorder, the eventual diagnosis was paranoid schizophrenia. In recent years, the reverse situation occurs: Patients with what appears to be paranoid schizophrenia resistant to usual antipsychotic drugs may respond to lithium, and their conditions may be diagnosed retrospectively as manic-depressive disorder." Hollister, "Drugs for Emotional Disorders: Current Problems," *JAMA*, 234 (Dec. 1, 1975): 942–947; quote, p. 945. The classic German psychopathologists, however, were quite aware that a "schizophrenia" diagnosis could be a mood disorder or catatonia. See, for example, Oswald Bumke, *Lehrbuch der Geisteskrankheiten*, 2nd ed. (Munich: Bergmann, 1924), 611, 929, 934.

8. Harry J. Haynes and Chester L. Carlisle, "The Treatment of Schizophrenia with Desoxycorticosterone Acetate," *Medical Bulletin of the Veterans' Administration*, 18 (1941–1942): 141–147; quote, 145.

9. Max Reiss and Yolande M. L. Golla, "The Influence of the Endocrines on Cerebral Circulation," *Journal of Mental Science*, 86 (1940): 281–286.

10. R[obert] E. Hemphill and E[rwin] Stengel, "Morgagni's Syndrome: A Clinical and Pathological Study," *Journal of Mental Science*, 86 (1940): 341–365. See J. D. Fulton et al., "Hyperostosis Frontalis Interna, Acromegaly and Hyperprolactinaemia," *Postgraduate Medical Journal*, 66 (1990): 16–19.

11. R[obert] E. Hemphill, "Hyperthyrotic Catatonia: A Schizophrenic Symptom-Complex," *Journal of Mental Science*, 88 (1942): 1–30. Gjessing briefly summarized his own work in "Disturbances of Somatic Functions in Catatonia with a Periodic Course, and Their Compensation," *Journal of Mental Science*, 84 (1938): 608–621.

12. R[obert] Hemphill, "Endocrinology in Clinical Psychiatry," *Journal of Mental Science*, 90 (1944): 410–434; quote, 417.

13. Ibid., 421, 423, 425, 428.

14. On "nonmelancholic depression," see Gordon Parker and Dusan Hadzi-Pavlovic, "A Clinical Algorithm for Defining Melancholia: Sub-typing Measures," in *Melancholia: A Disorder of Movement and Mood*, ed. Parker and Hadzi-Pavlovic (Cambridge, U.K.: Cambridge University Press, 1996), 202–210. The term "melancholic mood disorder" is suggested by Edward Shorter, "The Doctrine of the Two Depressions in Historical Perspective," in *Melancholia: Beyond DSM, Beyond Neurotransmitters*, ed. Tom Bolwig and Edward Shorter, *Acta Psychiatrica Scandinavica Supplementum*, 115, no. 433 (2007): 7–13.

15. G. Tayleur Stockings, "A New Euphoriant for Depressive Mental States," *BMJ*, 1 (June 28, 1947): 918–922. His remedy of choice was not an adrenocorticoid but Synhexyl, a cannabinoid recently synthesized by Roche.

16. Bernard J. Carroll, "Psychopathology and Neurobiology of Manic-Depressive Disorders," in *Psychopathology and the Brain*, ed. B. J. Carroll and J. E. Barrett (New York: Raven Press), 265–285.

17. Donald F. Klein and John M. Davis, *Diagnosis and Drug Treatment* (Baltimore: Williams & Wilkins, 1969).

18. Hans Selye, *The Stress of My Life: A Scientist's Memoirs* (New York: Van Nostrand, 1979), 60.

19. Hans Selye, "A Syndrome Produced by Diverse Nocuous Agents," *Nature*, 138 (July 4, 1936): 32.

20. W[alter] B. Cannon, "The Interrelations of Emotions as Suggested by Recent Physiological Researches," *American Journal of Physiology*, 25 (1914): 256–282. For example: "At times of stress, blood may be driven out of vegetative organs of the interior, which serve the routine needs of the body, into the skeletal muscles . . . ." (p. 269) He introduces the concept of "flight or fight" in this article.

21. Hans Selye, *The Physiology and Pathology of Exposure to Stress: A Treatise Based on the Concepts of the General-Adaptation-Syndrome and the Diseases of Adaptation* (Montreal: Acta, 1950), 3.

22. Jan A. Fawcett and William E. Bunney, Jr., "Pituitary Adrenal Function and Depression," *Archives of General Psychiatry*, 16 (1967): 517–535. They claim that psychiatric interest in pituitary and adrenal function began with Selye (p. 517).

23. Roger Guillemin, "Pioneering in Neuroendocrinology 1952–1969," in *Pioneers in Neuroendocrinology II*, ed. Joseph Meites, Bernard T. Donovan, and Samuel M. McCann (New York: Plenum, 1978), 221–239; quote, 224.

24. Seymour Levine, "Discussion: Stress," in *Neuroendocrinology and Psychiatric Disorder*, ed. Gregory M. Brown, Stephen H. Koslow, and Seymour Reichlin (New York: Raven, 1984), 145–150; quote, 146.

25. A[lois] E. Kornmüller, "Der Mechanismus des epileptischen Anfalles auf Grund bioelektrischer Untersuchungen am Zentralnervensystem," *Fortschritte der Neurologie und Psychiatrie*, 7 (1935): 391–400, 414–432. See also Frederic A. Gibbs, William G. Lennox, and Erna L. Gibbs, "The Electro-encephalogram in Diagnosis and in Localization of Epileptic Seizures," *AMA Archives of Neurology and Psychiatry*, 36 (1936): 1225–1235. For a brief overview of Berger and his work, see Edward Shorter, *Historical Dictionary of Psychiatry* (New York: Oxford University Press, 2005), 42.

26. W. Zimmermann, "Eine Farbreaktion der Sexualhormone und ihre Anwendung zur quantitativen colorimetrischen Bestimmung," *Hoppe-Seyler's Zeitschrift für physiologische Chemie*, 233 (1935): 257–264.

27. N[ancy] H[elen] Callow et al., "Methods of Extracting Compounds Related to the Steroid Hormones from Human Urine," *Journal of Endocrinology*, 1 (1939): 76–98.

28. M[ax] Reiss et al., "Regulation of Urinary Steroid Excretion: 1. Effects of Dehydro*iso*androsterone and of Anterior Pituitary Extract on the Pattern of Daily Excretion in Man," *Biochemical Journal*, 44 (1949): 632–635. Dehydro*epi*androsterone has become the more familiar term for their dehydro*iso*androsterone. The exact urinary metabolite they studied was 3(alpha)-hydroxy-ketosteroid.

29. J[ohan] H. W. van Ophuijsen, "A New Phase in Clinical Psychiatry, Part I and Introduction: Endocrinologic Orientation to Psychiatric Disorders," *Journal of Clinical and Experimental Psychopathology*, 12 (1951): 1–4; quote, 2.

30. Arthur M. Sackler, Raymond R. Sackler, Félix Marti-Ibáñez, and Mortimer D. Sackler, "Contemporary Physiodynamic Trends in Psychiatry," *Journal of Clinical and Experimental Psychopathology and Quarterly Review of Psychiatry and Neurology*, 15 (1954): 382–400; see esp. 389–390.

31. Oldrich Vinar, "The Neurotransmitter Era in Psychopharmacology: Reflections of a Clinician," in *The Neurotransmitter Era in Neuropsychopharmacology*, ed. Thomas A. Ban and Ronaldo Ucha Udabe (Buenos Aires: Polemos, 2006), 201–210; see esp. 201.

32. J[ames] B. Collip, Evelyn B. Anderson, and D. L. Thomson, "The Adrenotropic Hormone of the Anterior Pituitary Lobe," *Lancet*, 2 (Aug. 12, 1933): 347–348.

33. Choh Hao Li, Herbert M. Evans, and Miriam E. Simpson, "Adrenocorticotropic Hormone," *Journal of Biological Chemistry*, 149 (1943): 413–424.

34. William F. Ganong, "The Brain and the Endocrine System: A Memoir," in *Pioneers in Neuroendocrinology* (Meites), 189–200; see esp. 191.

35. Howard P. Rome and Francis J. Braceland, "The Psychological Response to ACTH, Cortisone, Hydrocortisone and Related Steroid Substances," *AJP*, 108 (1951–52): 641–651; quote, 647.

36. I. Arthur Mirsky, Robert Miller, and Marvin Stein, "Relation of Adrenocortical Activity and Adaptive Behavior," *Psychosomatic Medicine*, 15 (1953): 574–588.

37. See Leo Alexander, *Treatment of Mental Disorder* (Philadelphia: Saunders, 1953), 312, 459–460, who found it unpromising as a treatment. Investigators at Mt. Sinai Hospital in New York found that ACTH and cortisone induced mental symptoms rather than relieving them. Paul Goolker and Joseph Schein, "Psychic Effects of ACTH and Cortisone," *Psychosomatic Medicine*, 15 (1953): 589–613.

38. M[ax] Reiss et al., "Adrenocortical Responsivity in Relation to Psychiatric Illness and Treatment with ACTH and ECT," *Journal of Clinical and Experimental Psychopathology*, 12 (1951): 171–182; quote, 173.

39. Dwight J. Ingle, "Edward C. Kendall: March 8, 1886–May 4, 1972," *Biographical Memoirs, National Academy of Sciences (U.S.)*, 47 (1974): 249–290; see esp. 267.

40. Lewis Hastings Sarett, "Partial Synthesis . . . ," *Journal of Biological Chemistry*, 162 (1946): 601–631.

41. Ingle, "Kendall," 271.

42. C[harles] W. Shoppee, "The Chemistry of Cortisone," *Annual Review of Biochemistry*, 22 (1953): 261–298, esp. 288–290.

43. N[orman] L. Wendler, R. P. Graber, R. E. Jones, and M. Tishler, "Synthesis of 11-Hydroxylated Cortical Steroids; 17-Alpha-Hydroxycorticosterone," letter, *Journal of the American Chemical Society*, 72 (1950): 5793–5794.

44. C. C. Porter and R. H. Silber, "A Quantitative Color Reaction for Cortisone and Related 17,21 Dihydroxy-20-Ketosteroids," *Journal of Biological Chemistry*, 185 (1950): 201–207.

45. Don H. Nelson and Leo T. Samuels, "A Method for the Determination of 17-Hydroxycorticosteroids in Blood: 17-Hydroxycorticosterone in Peripheral Circulation," *Journal of Clinical Endocrinology and Metabolism*, 12 (1952): 519–526. See also E. Myles Glenn and Don H. Nelson, "Chemical Method for the Determination of 17-Hydroxycorticosteroids and 17-Ketosteroids in Urine Following Hydrolysis with Beta-Glucuronidase," *Journal of Clinical Endocrinology and Metabolism*, 13 (1953): 911–921.

46. Eugene L. Bliss, Claude J. Migeon, C. H. Hardin Branch, and Leo T. Samuels, "Reaction of the Adrenal Cortex to Emotional Stress," *Psychosomatic Medicine*, 18 (1956): 56–76. The findings were first presented at a meeting of the American Psychosomatic Society on Mar. 27, 1954.

47. C. Kirschbaum, K. M. Pirke, and D. H. Hellhammar, "'The Trier Social Stress Test'—a Tool for Investigating Psychobiological Stress Response in a Laboratory Setting," *Neuropsychobiology*, 28 (1993): 76–81.

48. Diogo Furtado, "Les Rapports des thérapeutiques endocriniennes et vasomotrices in psychiatrie," in *Premier Congrès Mondial de Psychiatrie, Paris 1950*, vol. 4, ed. Henry Ey (Paris: Hermann, 1952), 457–471.

49. R[obert] E. Hemphill and M[ax] Reiss, "A.C.T.H. in Psychiatry," ibid., 471–480.

50. Léon Fouks et al., "Treatment of Acute and Chronic Schizophrenic States," in *Psychopharmacology Frontiers: Proceedings of the Psychopharmacology Symposium, Second International Congress of Psychiatry*, ed. Nathan S. Kline (Boston: Little, Brown [1957]), 127–132; quote, 130. They wrote "androstalolon," an evident typo for androstanolone (stanolone).

51. Hudson Hoagland, discussion, in *Hormones, Brain Function, and Behavior: Proceedings of a Conference on Neuroendocrinology Held at Arden House, Harriman, New York, 1956*, ed. Hoagland (New York: Academic, 1957), 21. This bioethically interesting episode has gone widely unnoticed by historians of medicine.

52. See "1958 Corticosteroid Competition," *F-D-C Reports/Pink Sheet* (March 9, 1959): 8.

53. Francis Board, Harold Persky, and David A. Hamburg, "Psychological Stress and Endocrine Functions: Blood Levels of Adrenocortical and Thyroid Hormones in Acutely Disturbed Patients," *Psychosomatic Medicine*, 18 (1956): 324–333. Persky is identified as a Ph.D. and may have supervised the tests. The findings were first presented at the annual meeting of the American Psychosomatic Society, May 4, 1955. This project produced several articles, including this one by Francis Board, Ralph Wadeson, and Harold Persky, "Depressive Affect and Endocrine Functions," *AMA Archives of Neurology and Psychiatry*, 78 (1957): 612–620.

54. Douglas B. Price, M. Thaler, and J. W. Mason don't cite the Board-Hamburg research, but essentially replicate it: "Preoperative Emotional States and Adrenal Cortical Activity," *AMA Archives of Neurology and Psychiatry*, 77 (1957): 646–656. They offer one of the first indications, moreover, that cortisol levels are normal in "schizophrenia" (or at least among supposed schizophrenics awaiting cardiac or pulmonary surgery, their study group).

55. Ralph E. Peterson, Aurora Karrer, and Serafim L. Guerra, "Evaluation of Silber-Porter Procedure for Determination of Plasma Hydrocortisone," *Analytical Chemistry*, 29 (1957): 144–149; C. B. Hatfield and S. Shuster, "The Inhibitory Effect of Triamcinolone on Adrenal Function," *Journal of Clinical Pathology*, 12 (1959): 140–142. The revised Silber-Porter reaction, described in 1954, was highly specific for cortisol. Robert H. Silber and Curt C. Porter, "The Determination of 17,21-Dihydroxy-20-Ketosteroids in Urine and Plasma," *Journal of Biological Chemistry*, 210 (1954): 923–932. On changes in the measurement of adrenal corticosteroids, see Richard P. Michael and James L. Gibbons, "Interrelationships Between the Endocrine System and Neuropsychiatry," *International Review of Neurobiology*, 5 (1963): 243–302; see esp. 247.

56. James L. Gibbons and Paul R. McHugh, "Plasma Cortisol in Depressive Illness," *Journal of Psychiatric Research*, 1 (1962): 162–171.

57. Paul McHugh interview, by Max Fink, Stony Brook, N.Y, Dec. 10, 2007.

58. Howard D. Kurland, "Steroid Excretion in Depressive Disorders," *Archives of General Psychiatry*, 10 (1964): 554–560.

59. Howard D. Kurland, "Physiologic Treatment of Depressive Reactions: A Pilot Study," *AJP*, 122 (1965): 457–458.

60. Robert T. Rubin and Arnold J. Mandel, "Adrenal Cortical Activity in Pathological Emotional States: A Review," *AJP*, 123 (1966): 387–400.

61. See David A. Hamburg, "Adult Psychiatry Research at the NIMH in the 1950s," in *Mind, Brain, Body, and Behavior: Foundations of Neuroscience and Behavioral Research at the National Institutes of Health*, ed. Ingrid G. Farreras, Caroline Hannaway, and Victoria A. Harden (Amsterdam: IOS Press, 2004), 245–256.

62. Ibid., 248.

63. Ibid., 249.

64. William E. Bunney, Jr., John W. Mason, John F. Roatch, and David A. Hamburg, "A Psychoendocrine Study of Severe Psychotic Depressive Crises," *AJP*, 122 (1965): 72–80.

65. William E. Bunney, Jr., and Jan A. Fawcett, "Possibility of a Biochemical Test for Suicidal Potential: An Analysis of Endocrine Findings Prior to Three Suicides," *Archives of General Psychiatry*, 13 (1965): 232–239; see also William E. Bunney, Jr., and Jan A. Fawcett, "Biochemical Research in Depression and Suicide," in *Suicidal Behaviors: Diagnosis and Management*, ed. H. L. P. Resnik (Boston: Little Brown, 1968), 145–159.

66. Jan A. Fawcett and William E. Bunney, Jr., "Pituitary Adrenal Function and Depression: An Outlook for Research," *Archives of General Psychiatry*, 16 (1967): 517–535; quote, 518. See also William E. Bunney, Jr., Jan A. Fawcett, J. M. Davis, and S. Gifford, "Further Evaluation of Urinary 17-Hydroxycorticosteroids in Suicidal Patients," *Archives of General Psychiatry*, 21 (1969): 138–150.

67. *Recent Advances in the Psychobiology of the Depressive Illnesses: Proceedings of a Workshop Sponsored by the Clinical Research Branch, Division of Extramural Research Programs, National Institute of Mental Health*, ed. Thomas A. Williams, Martin M. Katz, and James Asa Shield, Jr. (Washington, D.C.: GPO, 1972; DHEW Pub. No. [HSM] 70–9053).

68. Ronald De Kloet, G. Wallach, and B. S. McEwen, "Differences in Corticosterone and Dexamethasone Binding to Rat Brain and Pituitary," *Endocrinology*, 96 (1975): 598–609; Maureen E. Keller-Wood and M. F. Dallman, "Corticosteroid Inhibition of ACTH Secretion," *Endocrine Reviews*, 5 (1984): 1–24.

69. Grant W. Liddle, "Tests of Pituitary-Adrenal Suppressibility in the Diagnosis of Cushing's Syndrome," *Journal of Clinical Endocrinology and Metabolism*, 20 (1960): 1539–1560.

70. J[ames] L. Gibbons and T. J. Fahy, "Effect of Dexamethasone on Plasma Corticosteroids in Depressive Illness," *Neuroendocrinology*, 1 (1966): 358–363.

71. Peter E. Stokes, "Pituitary Suppression in Psychiatric Patients," abstract no. 150, Endocrine Society, *Program of the Forty-Eighth Meeting* (1966): 101.

72. P. W. P. Butler and G. M[ichael] Besser, "Pituitary-Adrenal Function in Severe Depressive Illness," *Lancet*, 1 (June 8, 1968): 1234–1236.

73. Bernard Carroll, personal communication, July 31, 2007.

Notes to Chapter 4

1. Bernard J. Carroll, "Early Days in Melbourne: Reminiscences: Prepared for a History of the Department of Psychiatry, The University of Melbourne," ed. Edmond Chiu and Graham Burrows, 2008 (unpublished memoir supplied to the author by Carroll).

2. Alec Coppen, "The Biochemistry of Affective Disorders," *British Journal of Psychiatry*, 113 (1967): 1237–1264.

3. Information in these two paragraphs is owing to a private communication to the authors from Bernard Carroll, Aug. 2, 2007.

4. B[ernard] J. Carroll, F. I. R. Martin, and Brian Davies, "Resistance to Suppression by Dexamethasone of Plasma 11-O.H.C.S. Levels in Severe Depressive Illness," *BMJ*, 2 (Aug. 3, 1968): 285–287.

5. Paul McHugh, interview by Max Fink, Stony Brook, New York, Dec. 10, 2007.

6. James L. Gibbons, "Corticoid Metabolism in Depressive Illness," *Psychiatria, Neurologia, Neurochirurgia*, 72 (1969): 195–199; paper presented at the Symposium on Depression, Amsterdam, Sept. 27, 1968.

7. Arthur J. Prange, Jr., "Psychoendocrinology: A Commentary," *Psychoneuroendocrinology*, 21 (1998): 491–505; quote, 496.

8. Bernard J. Carroll et al., "A Specific Laboratory Test for the Diagnosis of Melancholia: Standardization, Validation, and Clinical Utility," *Archives of General Psychiatry*, 38 (1981): 15–22; see esp. 19.

9. Bernard J. Carroll, "Studies with Hypothalamic-Pituitary-Adrenal Stimulation Tests in Depression," in *Depressive Illness: Some Research Studies*, ed. Brian Davies, Bernard J. Carroll, and Robert M. Mowbray (Springfield, Ill.: Thomas, 1972), 149–201; see esp. 147.

10. Bernard J. Carroll, George C. Curtis and Joseph Mendels, "Neuroendocrine Regulation in Depression," *Archives of General Psychiatry*, 33 (1976): 1039–1044 and 1051–1058.

11. Ibid., 1051–1058.

12. This was the gist of Bernard J. Carroll's "The Hypothalamus-Pituitary-Adrenal Axis in Depression," in *Handbook of Studies on Depression*, ed. G. D. Burrows (Amsterdam: Excerpta Med, 1977), 325–342. The quoted sentence is from Carroll, "The Dexamethasone Suppression Test for Melancholia," *British Journal of Psychiatry*, 140 (1982): 292–304; see esp. 292.

13. B[ernard] J. Carroll, "Psychoendocrinology of Depression—Synopsis," paper delivered at 7th International Congress, International Society for Psychoneuroendocrinology, Strasbourg, France, July 13–16, 1976; Carroll Papers, International Psychopharmacology Archives, Eskind Biomedical Library, Vanderbilt University Medical Center, Nashville, Tenn.

14. Bernard Carroll, "Combining Laboratory and Clinical Criteria for Depression—This Week's Citation Classic," *Current Contents*, 32 (41) (Oct. 9, 1989): 14–15; quote, 14.

15. John F. Greden et al., "Normalization of Dexamethasone Suppression Test: A Laboratory Index of Recovery from Endogenous Depression," *Biological Psychiatry*, 15 (1980): 449–458.

16. See *Melancholia: A Disorder of Movement and Mood*, ed. Gordon Parker and Dusan Hadzi-Pavlovic (Cambridge, U.K.: Cambridge University Press, 1996).

17. Carroll in *Handbook* (ed. Burrows), 326.

18. Bernard J. Carroll et al., "Diagnosis of Endogenous Depression: Comparison of Clinical, Research and Neuroendocrine Criteria," *Journal of Affective Disorders*, 2 (1980): 177–194.

19. Bernard J. Carroll, "The Dexamethasone Suppression Test for Melancholia," *British Journal of Psychiatry*, 140 (1982): 292–304; see Table 1, p. 293.

20. Bernard Carroll, personal communication to Edward Shorter, Feb. 28, 2006.

21. Carroll, "Specific Laboratory Test" (1981); quotes, 15, 20, 22.

22. Carroll, in *Handbook* (ed. Burrows), 339.

23. Mihaly Aratò, "Back and Forth to the Future," in *From Psychopharmacology to Neuropsychopharmacology in the 1980s*, ed. Thomas A. Ban, David Healy, and Edward Shorter (Budapest: Animula, 2002), 140–143; quote, 141.

24. Robert Rubin interview by Edward Shorter and Max Fink, Hollywood, Fla., Dec. 5, 2006.

25. McHugh–Fink interview, 2007.

26. Bernard J. Carroll, John F. Greden, and Michael Feinberg, "Neuroendocrine Disturbances and the Diagnosis and Aetiology of Endogenous Depression," *Lancet*, 1 (1980): 321–322.

27. David Sachar, one-page memoir, attached to an e-mail from David Sachar to Edward Shorter, Aug. 6, 2007.

28. Marvin Stein interview by Edward Shorter and Max Fink, New York City, Oct. 24, 2007.

29. McHugh–Fink interview, 2007.

30. Edward Sachar to "Dear Folks," Aug. 4 [1959]; Abram Sachar Personal Papers Collection, Brandeis University Archives, Waltham, Mass.

31. John W. Mason et al., "The Role of Limbic System Structures in the Regulation of ACTH Secretion," *Acta Neurovegetativa*, 23 (1961): 4–14. We are grateful to Rachel Yarmolinsky of the New York State Psychiatric Institute for a copy of Sachar's bibliography.

32. Edward J. Sachar, "Now Is the Summer of Our Discontent," *Harvard Medical Alumni Bulletin*, Fall, 1964, pagination missing.

33. These details are primarily from an obituary in the *New York Times* (March 28, 1984): B4.

34. Joseph H. Handlon et al., "Psychological Factors Lowering Plasma 17-Hydroxycorticosteroid Concentration," *Psychosomatic Medicine*, 24 (1962): 535–542.

35. Edward J. Sachar, John W. Mason, Harold S. Kolmer, Jr., and Kenneth L. Artiss, "Psychoendocrine Aspects of Acute Schizophrenic Reactions," *Psychosomatic Medicine*, 25 (1963): 510–537; quote, 510.

36. Edward J. Sachar J. M. Mackenzie, W. A. Binstock, and J. E. Mack, "Corticosteroid Responses to Psychotherapy of Depressions, I: Evaluations During Confrontation of Loss," *Archives of General Psychiatry*, 16 (1967): 461–470.

37. Edward J. Sachar, S. S. Kantner, D. Buie, et al., "Psychoendocrinology of Ego Disintegration," *AJP*, 126 (1970): 1067–1078.

38. Edward J. Sachar, Leon Hellman, Thomas F. Gallagher, and David K. Fukushima, "Cortisol Production in Depressions," in *Recent Advances in the Psychobiology of the Depressive Illnesses: Proceedings of a Workshop Sponsored by the Clinical Research Branch, Division of Extramural Research Programs, National Institute of Mental Health*, ed. Thomas A. Williams, Martin M. Katz, and James Asa Shield, Jr. (Washington, D.C.: GPO, 1972; DHEW Pub. No. [HSM] 70–9053), 221–228.

39. Edward J. Sachar, Leon Hellman, David K. Fukushima, and Thomas F. Gallagher, "Cortisol Production in Depressive Illness: A Clinical and Biochemical Clarification," *Archives of General Psychiatry*, 23 (1970): 289–298.

40. Ibid.; quote, 298.

41. Edward J. Sachar, Leon Hellman, David K. Fukushima, and Thomas F. Gallagher, "Cortisol Production in Mania," *Archives of General Psychiatry*, 26 (1972): 137–139.

42. Herbert Y. Meltzer, Edward J. Sachar, and Andrew G. Frantz, "Serum Prolactin Levels in Unmedicated Schizophrenic Patients," *Archives of General Psychiatry*, 31 (1974): 564–569.

43. Edward J. Sachar, Jordan Finkelstein, and Leon Hellman, "Growth Hormone Responses in Depressive Illness," *Archives of General Psychiatry*, 25 (1971): 263–269.

44. B[ernard] J. Carroll, "Hypothalamic-Pituitary Function in Depressive Illness: Insensitivity to Hypoglycaemia," *BMJ*, 3 (5 July 1969): 27–28.

45. Edward J. Sachar, Andrew G. Frantz, Norman Altman, and Jon Sassin, "Growth Hormone and Prolactin in Unipolar and Bipolar Depressed Patients: Responses to Hypoglycemia and L-Dopa," *AJP*, 130 (1973): 1362–1367.

46. Edward J. Sachar et al., "Disrupted 24-Hour Patterns of Cortisol Secretion in Psychotic Depression," *Archives of General Psychiatry*, 28 (1973): 19–24; quote, 22.

47. David R. Rubinow et al., "The Relationship Between Cortisol and Clinical Phenomenology of Affective Illness," in *Neurobiology of Mood Disorders*, ed. Robert M. Post and James C. Ballenger (Baltimore: Williams & Wilkins, 1984), 271–289; quote, 280.

48. Edward J. Sachar, Andrew G. Frantz, Norman Altman, and Jon Sassin, "Growth Hormone and Prolactin in Unipolar and Bipolar Depressed Patients: Responses to Hypoglycemia and L-Dopa," *AJP*, 130 (1973): 362–366.

49. Ibid.; quote, 365.

50. Peter H. Gruen, Edward J. Sachar, Norman Altman, and Jon Sassin, "Growth Hormone Responses to Hypoglycemia in Postmenopausal Depressed Women," *Archives of General Psychiatry*, 32 (1975): 31–33; quote, 31.

51. Joseph J. Schildkraut, "The Catecholamine Hypothesis of Affective Disorders: A Review of Supporting Evidence," *AJP*, 122 (1965): 509–522.

52. Robert M. Rose, discussion, in *Neuroendocrinology and Psychiatric Disorder*, ed. Gregory M. Brown, Stephen H. Koslow, and Seymour Reichlin (New York: Raven, 1984), 91. The symposium took place in 1983.

53. Bernard J. Carroll and Joseph Mendels, "Neuroendocrine Regulation in Affective Disorders," in *Hormones, Behavior and Psychopathology*, ed. Edward J. Sachar (New York: Raven Press, 1976), 193–224; quote, 218.

54. Edward J. Sachar et al., "Use of Neuroendocrine Techniques in Psychopharmacological Research," in *Hormones, Behavior and Psychopathology* (ed. Sachar), 161–176.

55. Edward J. Sachar, Peter H. Gruen, and Norman Altman, "The Use of the Prolactin Response in Clinical Psychopharmacology," *Psychopharmacology Bulletin*, 13 (1977): 60–61.

56. Sachar, *Hormones, Behavior and Psychopathology;* the meeting took place in March 1975.

57. Uriel Halbreich interview with Edward Shorter and Max Fink, Dec. 4, 2006, Hollywood, Fla.

58. This work is mentioned in Sachar, "Neuroendocrine Techniques," *Hormones, Behavior and Psychopathology*, 161–176; see esp. 162–163.

59. Edward J. Sachar et al., "Dextroamphetamine and Cortisol in Depression: Morning Plasma Cortisol Levels Suppressed," *Archives of General Psychiatry*, 37 (1980): 755–757.

60. Edward. J. Sachar et al., "Paradoxical Cortisol Responses to Dextroamphetamine in Endogenous Depression," *Archives of General Psychiatry*, 38 (1981): 1113–1117.

61. Edward J. Sachar et al., "Three Tests of Cortisol Secretion in Adult Endogenous Depressives," *Acta Psychiatrica Scandinavica*, 71 (1985): 1–8.

62. Gregory M. Asnis et al., "Plasma Cortisol Secretion and REM Period Latency in Adult Endogenous Depression," *AJP*, 140 (1983): 750–753.

63. Edward J. Sachar and Miron Baron, "The Biology of Affective Disorders," *Annual Review of Neuroscience*, 2 (1979): 505–518; quote, 517.

64. McHugh–Fink interview, 2007.

Notes to Chapter 5

1. *Depressive Illness: Some Research Studies*, ed. Brian Davies, Bernard J. Carroll, and Robert M. Mowbray (Springfield, Ill.: Thomas, 1972).

2. Edward J. Sachar et al., "Use of Neuroendocrine Techniques in Psychopharmacological Research," in *Hormones, Behavior, and Psychopathology*, ed. Sachar (New York: Raven, 1976), 161–176.

3. Walter Brown interview with Edward Shorter and Max Fink, Feb. 16, 2006, at Tiverton, R.I.

4. George Arana, interview with Max Fink, Jan. 4, 2006, in Charleston, S.C.

5. Robert M. Rose, discussion, in *Neuroendocrinology and Psychiatric Disorder*, ed. Gregory M. Brown, Stephen H. Koslow, and Seymour Reichlin (New York: Raven, 1984), 226; the symposium occurred in 1983.

6. Michael Schlesser, George Winokur, and Barry M. Sherman, "Hypothalamic-Pituitary-Adrenal Axis Activity in Depressive Illness: Its Relationship to Classification," *Archives of General Psychiatry*, 37 (1980): 737–743.

7. Dwight Landis Evans and Charles B. Nemeroff, "The Dexamethasone Suppression Test in Mixed Bipolar Disorder," *AJP*, 140 (1983): 615–617.

8. Zoltán Rihmer, Erika Szádoczky and Mihály Arató, "Dexamethasone Suppression Test in Masked Depression," *Journal of Affective Disorders*, 5 (1983): 293–296.

9. C. M. Banki et al., "Associations Among Dexamethasone Non-suppression and TRH-Induced Hormonal Responses: Increased Specificity for Melancholia?" *Psychoneuroendocrinology*, 11 (1986): 205–211.

10. Mark Zimmerman, William Coryell, and Bruce Pfohl, "The Validity of the Dexamethasone Suppression Test as a Marker for Endogenous Depression," *Archives of General Psychiatry*, 43 (1986): 347–355; quotes, 352.

11. Dwight Landis Evans and Charles B. Nemeroff, "The Clinical Use of the Dexamethasone Suppression Test in DSM-III Affective Disorders: Correlation with the Severe Depressive Subtypes of Melancholia and Psychosis," *Journal of Psychiatric Research*, 21 (1987): 185–194; see Table 1, p. 188. The difference among results was also highly significant.

12. Kevin B. Miller and J. Craig Nelson, "Does the Dexamethasone Suppression Test Relate to Subtypes, Factors, Symptoms, or Severity?" *Archives of General Psychiatry*, 44 (1987): 769–774.

13. Walter A. Brown, G. Keitner, C. B. Qualls, amd R. Haier, "The Dexamethasone Suppression Test and Pituitary-Adrenocortical Function," *Archives of General Psychiatry*, 42 (1985): 121–123.

14. John J. Worthington to Walter A. Brown, Feb. 11, 1985, letter in Brown's private archive, Tiverton, R.I.

15. Walter Brown, "What Happened to the DST? This Week's Citation Classic," *Current Contents*, nos. 52–53 (Dec. 24–31, 1990): 12–13; quote, 13.

16. V. H. Asfeldt, "Simplified Dexamethasone Suppression Test," *Acta Endocrinologica*, 61 (1969): 219–231.

17. N. Herring and D. J. Paterson, "ECG Diagnosis of Acute Ischaemia and Infarction: Past, Present and Future," *Quarterly Journal of Medicine*, 99 (2006): 219–230; quote, 228.

18. Constance D. Lehman et al., "MRI Evaluation of the Contralateral Breast in Women with Recently Diagnosed Breast Cancer," *New England Journal of Medicine*, 356 (March 29, 2007): 1295–1303.

19. Max Fink, "Should the Dexamethasone Suppression Test Be Resurrected?" *Acta Psychiatrica Scandinavica*, 112 (2005): 245–249.

20. Bernard J. Carroll, discussion, in *Neuroendocrinology and Psychiatric Disorder* (ed. Brown), 283.

21. Peter E. Stokes, Peter M. Stoll, Marlin R. Mattson, and Robert N. Sollod, "Diagnosis and Psychopathology in Psychiatric Patients Resistant to Dexamethasone," in *Hormones, Behavior, and Psychopathology* (ed. Sachar), 225–229.

22. Eric D. Peselow et al., "Plasma Cortisol Values after Dexamethasone in Depressed Inpatients," *Journal of Clinical Psychopharmacology*, 3 (1983): 45–46.

23. Ru-Band Lu, Swui-Ling Ho, Huei-Chen Huang, and Yu-Tsai Lin, "The Specificity of the Dexamethasone Suppression Test in Endogenous Depressive Patients," *Neuropsychopharmacology*, 1 (1988): 157–162.

24. George W. Arana, Robert J. Workman, and Ross J. Baldessarini, "Association Between Low Plasma Levels of Dexamethasone and Elevated Levels of Cortisol in Psychiatric Patients Given Dexamethasone," *AJP*, 141 (1984): 1619–1620; quotes, 1620.

25. R. E. Kendell et al., "Diagnostic Criteria of American and British Psychiatrists," *Archives of General Psychiatry*, 25 (1971):123–130; see Table 5, p. 127.

26. George Winokur and Paula Clayton, "Family History Studies: I. Two Types of Affective Disorders Separated According to Genetic and Clinical Factors," in *Recent Advances in Biological Psychiatry*, vol. 9, ed. J[oseph] Wortis (New York: Plenum, 1967), 35–50.

27. Eli Robins and Samuel B. Guze, "Establishment of Diagnostic Validity in Psychiatric Illness: Its Application to Schizophrenia," *AJP*, 126 (1970): 983–987.

28. Richard Abrams and Michael Alan Taylor, "Catatonia: A Prospective Clinical Study," *Archives of General Psychiatry*, 33 (1976): 579–581.

29. Robert L. Spitzer et al., "Preliminary Report of the Reliability of Research Diagnostic Criteria Applied in Psychiatric Case Records," in *Predictability in Psychopharmacology: Preclinical and Clinical Correlations*, ed. Abraham Sudilovsky, Samuel Gershon, and Bernard Beer (New York: Raven, 1975), 1–47. On the origins of *DSM-III*, see Edward Shorter, *Before Prozac: The Troubled History of Mood Disorders in Psychiatry* (New York: Oxford University Press, 2009).

30. American Psychiatric Association, *DSM-II: Diagnostic and Statistical Manual of Mental Disorders*, 2nd ed. (Washington, D.C.: American Psychiatric Association, 1968).

31. On the dynamics of the task force that produced this historic result, see Shorter, *Before Prozac*.

32. James R. Hodge, "The Whiplash Neurosis," *Psychosomatics*, 12 (1971): 245–249; quote, 245.

32. Gordon Parker, "Beyond Major Depression," *Psychological Medicine*, 35 (2005): 467–474; quotes, 467.

34. Max Fink and Robert Spitzer, discussion, in *Critical Issues in Psychiatric Diagnosis*, ed. Robert L. Spitzer and Donald F. Klein (New York: Raven, 1978), 334.

35. Among the oldest biological tests in psychiatry, the use of chemical agents to induce panic in those who are panic-prone was first described by Stanley Cobb and Mandel E. Cohen, "Experimental Production During Rebreathing of Sighing Respiration and Symptoms Resembling Those in Anxiety Attacks in Patients with Anxiety Neurosis," *Journal of Clinical Investigation*, 19 (1940): 789. On lactate, see F. N. Pitts and J. N. McClure, "Lactate Metabolism in Anxiety Neurosis," *New England Journal of Medicine*, 277 (1967): 1329–1336. See also Desmond Kelly, N. Mitchell-Heggs, and D. Sherman, "Anxiety and the Effects

of Sodium Lactate Assessed Clinically and Physiologically," *British Journal of Psychiatry*, 119 (1971); 129–141.

36. Robert Spitzer, interview by Edward Shorter and Max Fink, Mar. 14, 2007, at the Spitzer home in Irvington, N.Y.

37. Paul McHugh interview by Max Fink, Stony Brook, N.Y., Dec. 10, 2007.

38. Bernard Carroll, discussion, in *The Validity of Psychiatric Diagnosis*, ed. Lee N. Robins and James E. Barrett (New York: Raven, 1989), 303–304.

39. Bernard J. Carroll, "Combining Laboratory and Clinical Criteria for Depression: This Week's Citation Classic," *Current Contents*, 32 (41) (Oct. 9, 1989): 14–15; quote, 14.

40. World Health Organization, *Manual of the International Statistical Classification of Diseases, Injuries, and Causes of Death, Based on the Recommendations of the Ninth Revision Conference, 1975* (Geneva: WHO, 1977), 2 vols.

41. Bernard Carroll, interview by Edward Shorter and Max Fink, part I , Oct. 17, 2005, Carmel, Calif.

42. Bernard J. Carroll, "Diagnostic Validity and Laboratory Studies: Rules of the Game," in *Validity of Psychiatric Diagnosis* (Robins and Barrett), 229–245; see Table 1, p. 233.

43. W[illiam] Coryell, "DST Abnormality as a Predictor of Course in Major Depression," *Journal of Affective Disorders*, 19 (1990): 163–169; quote, 165.

44. William Coryell and Michael Schlesser, "The Dexamethasone Suppression Test and Suicide Prediction," *AJP*, 158 (2001): 748–753. See also W. H. Norman et al., "The Dexamethasone Suppression Test and Completed Suicide," *Acta Psychiatrica Scandinavica*, 81 (1990): 120–125.

45. J. John Mann et al., "Can Biological Tests Assist Prediction of Suicide in Mood Disorders?" *International Journal of Neuropsychopharmacology*, 9 (2006): 465–474, finding that a prediction model requiring both DST and CSF 5-HIAA to be positive had a positive predictive value (PPV) of 23 percent in suicide. See also J[ussi] Jokinen, A[nna]-L[ena] Nordström, and P[eter] Nordström, "Hypothalamic-Pituitary Adrenal (HPA) Axis and Suicide Risk in Mood Disorders," *Journal of Affective Disorders*, 107 (2008): S65–66; Jussi Jokinen et al., "DST Non-Suppression Predicts Suicide After Attempted Suicide," *Psychiatry Research*, 150 (2007): 297–303.

46. Ivan K. Goldberg, "Dexamethasone Suppression Test as Indicator of Safe Withdrawal of Antidepressant Therapy," *Lancet*, 2 (Feb. 16, 1980): 376.

47. John F. Greden et al., "Normalization of Dexamethasone Suppression Test: A Laboratory Index of Recovery from Endogenous Depression," *Biological Psychiatry*, 15 (1980): 449–458; quote, 449.

48. Saulo C. M. Ribeiro, Rajiv Tanden, Leon Grunhaus, John F. Greden, "The DST as a Predictor of Outcome in Depression: A Meta-Analysis," *AJP*, 150 (1993): 1618–1629; quote, 1618.

49. W[alter] A. Brown et al., "DST Nonsuppression Predicts Poor Placebo Response in Depression," paper presented at the 16th International Congress of the International Society of Psychoneuroendocrinology, Kyoto, Japan, April, 1985; see also Walter A. Brown, Ram K. Shrivastava, and Mihaly Arato, "Pre-Treatment Pituitary-Adrenocortical Status and Placebo Response in Depression," *Psychopharmacology Bulletin*, 23 (1987): 155–159.

50. Eric D. Peselow et al., "The Dexamethasone Suppression Test and Response to Placebo," *Journal of Clinical Psychopharmacology*, 6 (1986): 286–291.

51. Personal communication, Bernard Carroll to Max Fink and Edward Shorter, March 1, 2006.

52. See W[alter] A. Brown, "Treatment Response in Melancholia," *Acta Psychiatrica Scandinavica Supplementum*, 115, no. 433 (2007): 125–129.

53. On the subject of side effects, Brown and co-workers discovered that 56 percent of nonsuppressors "developed intolerable side effects during treatment with fluvoxamine," while only 13 percent of the suppressors did so. Walter Armin Brown, Mihaly Arato, and Ram Shivastava, "Pituitary-Adrenocortical Hyperfunction and Intolerance to Fluvoxamine, a Selective Serotonin Uptake Inhibitor," *AJP*, 143 (1986): 88–90.

54. Z. Rihmer et al., "Dexamethasone Suppression Test as an Aid for Selection of Specific Antidepressant Drugs in Patients with Endogenous Depression," *Pharmacopsychiatry*, 18 (1985): 306–308.

55. Walter Armin Brown et al., "What Is Vital Depression (Endogenous Depression or Melancholia), and How Can It Be Reliably Assessed," *Psychopharmacology Bulletin*, 18 (1988): 84–86; quote, 85.

56. William H. Coryell and Mark Zimmerman, "HPA Axis Hyperactivity and Recovery from Functional Psychoses," *AJP*, 146 (1989): 473–477. See also Coryell, "Phenomenological Approaches to the Schizoaffective Spectrum," in *The Overlap of Affective and Schizophrenic Spectra*, ed. Andreas Marneros and Hagop S. Akiskal (New York: Cambridge University Press, 2007), 133–144, esp. Table 7.6, p. 141.

57. A. Ariav Albala, John F. Greden, J. Tarika, and Bernard J. Carroll, "Changes in Serial Dexamethasone Suppression Tests Among Unipolar Depressives Receiving Electroconvulsive Treatment," *Biological Psychiatry*, 16 (1981): 551–560.

58. McHugh–Fink interview, 2007.

59. A. John Rush et al., "Sleep EEG and Dexamethasone Suppression Test Findings in Outpatients with Unipolar Major Depressive Disorders," *Biological Psychiatry*, 17 (1982): 327–341.

60. A. John Rush, D. E. Giles, H. P. Roffwarg, and C. R. Parker, "The Dexamethasone Suppression Test in Patients with Mood Disorders," *Journal of Clinical Psychiatry*, 57 (1996): 470–484.

61. World Health Organization Collaborative Study, "The Dexamethasone Suppression Test in Depression," *BJP*, 150 (1987): 459–462.

62. Mihály Arató to Walter Brown, Aug. 21, 1985; Brown's private archive.

63. C. M. Banki, M[ihály] Arató, and Z. Rihmer, "Neuroendocrine Differences among Subtypes of Schizophrenic Disorder? An Investigation with the Dexamethasone Suppression Test," *Neuropsychobiology*, 11 (1984): 174–177. See also Filippo M. Ferro et al., "Clinical Outcome and Psychoendocrinological Findings in a Case of Lethal Catatonia," *Biological Psychiatry*, 30 (1991): 197–200.

64. Seymour Reichlin, discussion, in *Neuroendocrinology and Psychiatric Disorder* (Brown), 287.

Notes to Chapter 6

1. Walter Brown interview by Edward Shorter and Max Fink, Feb. 16, 2006, Tiverton, R.I.

2. Bernard Carroll interview by Edward Shorter and Max Fink, part II, Oct. 18, 2005, Carmel, Calif.

3. Brown–Shorter/Fink interview, 2006.

4. Thomas R. Insel et al., "The Dexamethasone Suppression Test in Patients with Primary Obsessive-Compulsive Disorder," *Psychiatry Research*, 6 (1982): 153–160.

See also Insel et al., "Biological Markers in Obsessive-Compulsive and Affective Disorders," *Journal of Psychiatric Research*, 18 (1984): 407–423.

5. M. Berger et al., "The Limited Utility of the Dexamethasone Suppression Test for the Diagnostic Process in Psychiatry," *British Journal of Psychiatry*, 145 (1984): 372–382; quote, 380.

6. William H. Nelson, "The Dexamethasone Suppression Test: Interaction of Diagnosis, Sex, and Age in Psychiatric Inpatients," *Biological Psychiatry*, 19 (1984): 1293–1304; quotes, 1300, 1301.

7. Matt T. Bianchi and Brian M. Alexander, "Evidence Based Diagnosis: Does the Language Reflect the Theory?" *BMJ*, 333 (Aug. 26, 2006): 442–445; quote, 442.

8. Personal communication, Bernard Carroll to Edward Shorter, Aug. 17, 2007. Marvin Minsky is a cognitive scientist at the Massachusetts Institute of Technology. When he said this is unknown.

9. Martin Bland, *An Introduction to Medical Statistics*, 3rd ed. (Oxford, U.K.: Oxford University Press, 2000), 87.

10. Shorter and Fink, Carroll interview, part I, Oct. 17, 2005.

11. Bernard J. Carroll, "Dexamethasone Suppression Test: A Review of Contemporary Confusion," *Journal of Clinical Psychiatry*, 46 (1985): 13–24; quote, 13.

12. Brown–Shorter/Fink interview, 2006.

13. The criteria for endogenous depression or melancholia were presented in Bernard J Carroll, Michael Feinberg, John F. Greden, et al., "Diagnosis of Endogenous Depression: Comparison of Clinical, Research and Neuroendocrine Criteria," *Jounal of Affective Disorders*, 2 (1980): 177–194.

14. Bernard Carroll marginalia, [Walter Brown], "The DST and Diagnosis" (Sept. 20, 1983): 8; in Carroll's private archive, Carmel, Calif.

15. Carroll–Shorter/Fink interview, I, 2005.

16. Ibid.

17. A copy of "Agenda: Workshop on the Clinical Utility of the Dexamethasone Suppression Test," has been preserved in the archives of the American Psychiatric Association, Arlington, Va., Harold Pincus, Office of Research, box 15.

18. Undated memo in Carroll's handwriting, later confirmed by Carroll as 1983, in Carroll Papers, Eskind Biomedical Library, Vanderbilt University Medical Center, Nashville, Tenn.

19. Alan F. Schatzberg, "Discussion of 'Controversies in Psychiatry': Depression in the Medically Ill, Sleep Disorders in the Elderly, and the DST," *Journal of Clinical Psychiatry*, 46 (1985): 30–31.

20. Judith Godwin Rabkin, Jonathan Stewart and Donald F. Klein, "Overview on the Relevance of the Dexamethasone Suppression Test to Differential Diagnosis," in National Institute of Mental Health, *Clinical Utility of the Dexamethasone Suppression Test: Proceedings of a National Institute of Mental Health Workshop* [July 20–21, 1982] (Rockville, Md.: U.S. Department of Health and Human Services, Public Health Service, Alcohol, Drug Abuse and Mental Health Administration, National Institute of Mental Health, DHHS Pub. No. [ADM] 85–1318, 1985), 12–33; quote, 31.

21. Peter Stokes, "DST Update: The Hypothalamic-Pituitary-Adrenocortical Axis and Affective Illness," *Biological Psychiatry*, 22 (1987): 245–248; quote, 246.

22. Steven D. Targum, "The Relevance of the Dexasmethasone Suppression Test to the Prediction of Treatment Response," in NIMH *Proceedings* (1982): 35–39; quote, 37–38.

23. Thomas R. Insel and Frederick K. Goodwin, "The Dexamethasone Suppression Test as a Predictor of Relapse," ibid., 41–43.

24. Thomas R. Insel and Frederick K. Goodwin, "The Dexamethasone Suppression Test: Promises and Problems of Diagnostic Laboratory Tests in Psychiatry," *Hospital and Community Psychiatry*, 34 (1983): 1131–1138; quote, 1135.

25. Thomas Insel to Alexander Glassman, Jan. 3, 1984; Walter Brown's private archive.

26. Herbert Y. Meltzer, "Factors Affecting the Validity of the Dexamethasone Suppression Test," NIMH *Proceedings* (1982): 54–57.

27. Brown–Shorter/Fink interview, 2006.

28. Carroll–Shorter/Fink interview, I, 2005. The authors interviewed Spitzer about these events but he could recall none of the details. Robert Spitzer interview by Edward Shorter and Max Fink, March 14, 2007, Irvington, N.Y.

29. Carroll–Shorter/Fink interview, 2005, part I.

30. Brown–Shorter/Fink interview, 2006.

31. NIMH *Proceedings* (1982).

32. Robert M. A. Hirschfeld, Stephen H. Koslow, and David J. Kupfer, "The Clinical Utility of the Dexamethasone Suppression Test in Psychiatry: Summary of a National Institute of Mental Health Workshop," *JAMA*, 250 (Oct. 28, 1983): 2172–2174; quotes, 2174. In response to several requests for an interview on various occasions, Hirschfeld claimed to have no time.

33. A. John Rush to Bernard Carroll, Jan. 24, 1983; Carroll Collection, International Neuropsychopharmacology Archives, Eskind Biomedical Library, Vanderbilt University Medical Center, Nashville, Tenn.

34. Stephen Sharfstein, Executive Member in Charge of Research, arrived at APA only in September of 1983. He has no recollection of the Task Force. Sharfstein to Edward Shorter, Apr. 10, 2006. Original APA documentation on its creation could not be found.

35. Harold Pincus, telephone interview with Max Fink, Apr. 10, 2006.

36. Ross J. Baldessarini, Seth Finklestein, and George W. Arana, "The Predictive Power of Diagnostic Tests and the Effect of Prevalence of Illness," *Archives of General Psychiatry*, 40 (1983): 569–573; quote, 573.

37. George Arana interview by Max Fink, Charleston, S.C., Jan. 4, 2006.

38. Bernard Carroll to Alexander H. Glassman, Oct. 24, 1983; Carroll's private archive.

39. See Brown to Glassman, June 4, 1984; in Brown's private archive.

40. George W. Arana, Robert J. Workman, and Ross J. Baldessarini, "Association Between Low Plasma Levels of Dexamethasone and Elevated Levels of Cortisol in Psychiatric Patients Given Dexamethasone," *AJP*, 141 (1984): 1619–1620.

41. Carroll, "DST: Contemporary Confusion."

42. Glassman to Brown, June 5, 1985; Brown's private archive.

43. Brown to Glassman, Sept. 16, 1985; Brown's private archive.

44. Council on Research, minutes, Sept. 19, 1985: 6; Office of Research, box 15, APA Archives.

45. George W. Arana, Ross J. Baldessarini and Marjorie Ornsteen, "The Dexamethasone Suppression Test for Diagnosis and Prognosis in Psychiatry," *Archives of General Psychiatry*, 42 (1985): 1193–1204; quote, 1201.

46. Carroll to Glassman, Dec. 29, 1985; Carroll's private archive.

47. Carroll to Glassman, Dec. 30, 1985; Carroll's private archive.

48. Carroll to Glassman, June 12, 1986; Carroll's private archive.

49. Glassman to Carroll (and Task Force), June 25, 1986; Carroll's private archive.

50. Carroll to Glassman, July 14, 1986; Carroll's private archive.

51. Harold Pincus's handwritten notes of the meeting, Sept. 10, 1986; Office of Research, box 15, APA Archives.

52. APA Task Force on Laboratory Tests in Psychiatry, "The Dexamethasone Suppression Test: An Overview of Its Current Status in Psychiatry," *AJP*, 144 (1987): 1253–1262; quote, 1259.

53. Ibid., 1259.

54. Ross Baldessarini interview with Edward Shorter and Max Fink, Feb. 17, 2006, McLean Hospital, Belmont, Mass.

55. Brown–Shorter/Fink interview, 2006.

56. Carroll–Shorter/Fink interview, I, 2005.

57. John Greden, interview by Thomas Ban, Dec. 7, 2003, San Juan, Puerto Rico.

58. Personal communication, Ross Baldessarini to Edward Shorter, Feb. 21, 2006.

59. Walter Brown, "What Happened to the DST? Citation Classic," *Current Contents*, 22 (52–53) (Dec. 24–31, 1990): 12–13; quote, 13.

60. Ibid., 12.

61. Robert Rubin interview by Edward Shorter and Max Fink, Dec. 5, 2006, Hollywood, Fla.

62. Baldessarini–Shorter/Fink interview, 2006.

63. Mihály Arató to Walter Brown, Sept. 14, 1986; Brown's private archive.

64. Carroll–Shorter/Fink interview, I, 2005.

65. Charles Nemeroff interview by Edward Shorter and Max Fink, Dec. 4, 2006, Hollywood, Fla.

66. Uriel Halbreich interview, by Edward Shorter and Max Fink, Dec. 4, 2006, Hollywood, Fla.

67. Carroll–Shorter/Fink interview, I, 2005.

68. Carroll to Donald Klein, June 26, 1997; in Carroll Collection, Archives, Eskind Memorial Library.

69. Michael Alan Taylor and Max Fink, *Melancholia: The Diagnosis, Pathophysiology, and Treatment of Depressive Illness* (New York: Cambridge University Press, 2006).

Notes to Chapter 7

1. Berta Scharrer, "Neurosecretion and Its Role in Neuroendocrine Regulation," in *Pioneers in Neuroendocrinology I*, ed. Joseph Meites, Bernard T. Donovan, and Samuel M. McCann (New York: Plenum, 1975), 257–265; quote, 257. The original publication was E[rnst] Scharrer, "Die Lichtempfindlichkeit blinder Elritzen (Untersuchungen über das Zwischenhirn der Fische I.)," *Zeitschrift für vergleichende Physiologie*, 7 (1928): 1–38.

2. Ernst Scharrer and Berta Scharrer, "Secretory Cells within the Hypothalamus," Association for Research in Nervous and Mental Disease, *Proceedings*, 20 (1939): 170–194.

3. Chandler M. Brooks, "Development of the Convergent Themes of Neuroendocrinology," in *Pioneers in Neuroendocrinology I* (ed. Meites), 63–79; quote, 65.

4. U[lf] von Euler and J[ohn] H. Gaddum, "An Unidentified Depressor Substance in Certain Tissue Extracts," *Journal of Physiology*, 72 (1931): 74–87.

5. Dorothy Price, "Feedback Control of Gonadal Hormones: Evolution of the Concept," in *Pioneers in Neuroendocrinology I* (ed. Meites), 219–238; quotes, 227, 228.

6. Carl R. Moore and Dorothy Price, "The Question of Sex Hormone Antagonism," *Proceedings of the Society for Experimental Biology and Medicine*, 28 (1930): 38–40.

7. Wolfgang Bargmann, "A Marvelous Region," in *Pioneers in Neuroendocrinology I* (ed. Meites), 37–43; quote, p. 39.

8. W[olfgang] Bargmann, "Über die neurosekretorische Verknüpfung von Hypotha-lamus und Neurohypophyse," *Zeitschrift für Zellforschung und Mikroskopische Anatomie,* 34 (1949): 610–634.

9. Brooks, in *Pioneers in Neuroendocrinology I (ed. Meites),* 70.

10. For a list of this research, see Marthe L. Vogt, "Geoffrey Wingfield Harris, 1913–1971," *Biographical Memoirs of Fellows of the Royal Society,* 18 (Nov. 1972): 309–329; bibliography begins at p. 322.

11. G[eoffrey] Raisman, "An Urge to Explain the Incomprehensible: Geoffrey Harris and the Discovery of the Neural Control of the Pituitary Gland," *Annual Review of Neuroscience,* 20 (1997): 533–566; quote, 537.

12. J[ohn] D[avis] Green and G[eoffrey] W. Harris, "Observation of the Hypophysio-Portal Vessels of the Living Rat," *Journal of Physiology,* 108 (1949): 359–361.

13. G[eoffrey] W. Harris and Dora Jacobsohn, "Proliferative Capacity of the Hypo-physial Portal Vessels," *Nature,* 165 (May 27, 1950): 854.

14. G[eoffrey] W. Harris and Dora Jacobsohn, "Functional Grafts of the Anterior Pituitary Gland," *Proceedings of the Royal Society of London,* ser. B, 139 (1951–52): 263–275; quote, 274. The paper was read in 1951, published in 1952.

15. J[acob] de Groot and G[eoffrey] W. Harris, "Hypothalamic Control of the Ante-rior Pituitary Gland and Blood Lymphocytes," *Journal of Physiology,* 111 (1950): 335–346.

16. Seymour Reichlin, "Formative Years as an Investigator of Hypothalamic-Pituitary Physiology," in *Pioneers in Neuroendocrinology II,* ed. Joseph Meites, Bernard T. Donovan, and Samuel M. McCann (New York: Plenum, 1978), 313–326; quote, 317.

17. G[eoffrey] W. Harris, *Neural Control of the Pituitary Gland* (London: Arnold, 1955), 165.

18. Murray Saffran and A[ndrew] V. Schally, "The Release of Corticotrophin by Anterior Pituitary Tissue in Vitro," *Canadian Journal of Biochemistry and Physiology,* 33 (1955): 408–415.

19. Murray Saffran, A[ndrew] V. Schally and B. G. Benfey, "Stimulation of the Release of Corticotropin From the Adenohypophysis By a Neurohypophyseal Factor," *Endocrinology,* 57 (1955): 439–444.

20. Roger Guillemin and Barry Rosenberg, "Humoral Hypothalamic Control of Anterior Pituitary: A Study with Combined Tissue Cultures," *Endocrinology,* 57 (1955): 599–607; quote, 606.

21. See Nicholas Wade, *The Nobel Duel: Two Scientists' 21-year Race to Win the World's Most Coveted Research Prize* (Garden City, N.Y.: Anchor, 1981), 20, 23.

22. See the table in *Pioneers in Neuroendocrinology II* (ed. Meites), 298.

23. Solomon A. Berson, Rosalyn S. Yalow, Arthur Bauman, et al., "Insulin-I[131] Metabolism in Human Subjects: Demonstration of Insulin Binding Globulin in the Circulation of Insulin Treated Subjects," *Journal of Clinical Investigation,* 35 (1956): 170–190.

24. The Nobel Prize in Physiology or Medicine 1977. Rosalyn Yalow, Autobiography. Available at http://www.nobelprize.org (accessed Aug. 26, 2007). See Rosalyn S. Yalow and Solomon A. Berson, "Assay of Plasma Insulin in Human Subjects by Immunological Methods," *Nature,* 184 (1959): 1648–1649. On the psychiatric nature of the patients, see Adolph Friedman, "Remembrance: The Berson and Yalow Saga," *Journal of Clinical Endocrinology & Metabolism,* 87 (2002): 1925–1928.

25. Edward Sachar to David Sachar, undated; on basis of internal evidence, evidently the summer of 1960. Abram Sachar Personal Papers Collection, Brandeis Uni-versity Archives, Waltham, Mass.

26. Interview with Walter A. Brown by Edward Shorter and Max Fink, Feb. 16, 2006, Tiverton, R.I.

27. Robert Rubin personal communication, Jan. 10, 2008.

28. Andrew V. Schally, "Aspects of Hypothalamic Regulation of the Pituitary Gland with Major Emphasis on Its Implications for the Control of Reproductive Processes," *Nobel Lectures, Physiology or Medicine, 1971–1980,* ed. Jan Lindsten (Singapore: World Scientific, 1992), 405–438; quote, 408.

29. Roger Guillemin, "Peptides in the Brain. The New Endocrinology of the Neuron," in *Nobel Lectures* (ed. Lindsten), 364–397; quote, 366. On the competition between Guillemin and Schally in the race to identify the hypothalamic releasing factors, see Wade, *Nobel Duel.*

30. Arthur J. Prange, Jr., "Psychoendocrinology: A Commentary," *Psychoneuroendocrinology,* 21 (1998): 491–505; quote, 495.

31. Dorothy T. Krieger and Howard P. Krieger, "Circadian Pattern of Plasma 17-Hydroxycorticosteroid: Alteration by Anticholinergic Agents," *Science,* 155 (March 17, 1967): 1421–1422; quote, 1422.

32. Eli Robins and Samuel B. Guze, "Establishment of Diagnostic Validity in Psychiatric Illness: Its Application to Schizophrenia," *AJP,* 126 (1970): 983–987; quote, 987.

33. David J. McClure and Robert A. Cleghorn, "Hormone Imbalance in Depressive States," in *The Future of the Brain Sciences: Proceedings of a Conference held at the New York Academy of Medicine, May 2–4, 1968,* ed. Samuel Bogoch (New York: Plenum, 1969), 525–553; quote, 530.

34. David A. Hamburg, "Projections for Future Research," in *Recent Advances in the Psychobiology of the Depressive Illnesses: Proceedings of a Workshop Sponsored by the Clinical Research Branch, Division of Extramural Research Programs, National Institute of Mental Health, Hosted by the College of William and Mary in Virginia, April 30 through May 2, 1969,* ed. Thomas A. Williams, Martin M. Katz, and James Asa Shield, Jr. (Washington, D.C.: GPO, 1972; DHEW Pub. No. [HSM] 70–9053), 351–355; quote, 353.

35. Edward J. Sachar et al., "Growth Hormone Responses in Depressive Illness," *Archives of General Psychiatry,* 25 (1971): 263–269.

36. J[ames] L. Gibbons, "Editorial: Endocrinology and Psychiatry," *Psychological Medicine,* 4 (1974): 240–243; quote, 242.

37. Gerhard Langer, G. Heinz, B. Reim, and Norbert Matussek, "Reduced Growth Hormone Responses to Amphetamine in 'Endogenous' Depressive Patients," *Archives of General Psychiatry,* 33 (1976): 1471–1475; quote, 1474.

38. Norbert Matussek, "Citation Classic: Alpha-$_2$-Adrenoceptor Subsensitivity in Depression," *Current Contents,* no. 32 (Aug. 7, 1989): 16. The research was published in Matussek et al., "Effect of Clonidine on Growth Hormone Release in Psychiatric Patients and Controls," *Psychiatric Research,* 2 (1980): 25–36.

39. Bernard J. Carroll, "Neuroendocrine Function in Psychiatric Disorders," in *Psychopharmacology: A Generation of Progress,* ed. Morris A. Lipton, Alberto DiMascio, and Keith F. Killam (New York: Raven, 1978), 487–497; quote, 487. The meeting was in 1976.

40. Jean Rossier, "From Neuropeptides to Neocortical Function: Path for Discoveries," in *Reflections on Twentieth-Century Psychopharmacology,* ed. Thomas A. Ban, David Healy, and Edward Shorter (Budapest: Animula, 2004), 361–367; quote, 362.

41. Peter C. Whybrow, "Studies in Thyroid and Brain: From Myxoedematosus Madness to Mood Modulation," in ibid., 510–516; quote, 512.

42. We are grateful to Dr. Prange for a copy of his curriculum vitae.

43. Thomas Ban, personal communication, Dec. 16, 2006.

44. Arthur J. Prange, Jr., "My Research in Psychothyroidology: An Autobiographical Note," in *The Triumph of Psychopharmacology*, ed. Thomas A. Ban, David Healy, and Edward Shorter (Budapest: Animula, 2000), 63–66; quote, 63.

45. Arthur J. Prange, Jr., Ian C. Wilson, Archie M. Rabon, and Morris A. Lipton, "Enhancement of Imipramine Antidepressant Activity by Thyroid Hormone," *AJP*, 126 (1969): 457–469.

46. Michael Posternak et al., "A Pilot Effectiveness Study: Placebo-Controlled Trial of Adjunctive L-triiodothyronine (T3) Used to Accelerate and Potentiate the Antidepressant Response," *International Journal of Neuropsychopharmacology*, 11 (2008): 15–25.

47. Peter C. Whybrow et al., "Thyroid Function and the Response of Liothyronine in Depression," *Archives of General Psychiatry*, 26 (1972): 242–245.

48. Prange, in *Triumph* (ed. Ban), 64.

49. A[lec] Coppen, D. M. Shaw, B. Herzberg, and R. Maggs, "Tryptophan in the Treatment of Depression," *Lancet*, 2 (1967): 1178–1180.

50. Bernard J. Carroll, Robert M. Mowbray, and Brian Davies, "Sequential Comparison of L-tryptophan with E.C.T. in Severe Depression," *Lancet*, 1 (May 9, 1970): 967–969.

51. U.S. Food and Drug Administration, Bureau of Drugs, Minutes of Neuropharmacology Advisory Committee meeting of Oct. 26, 1973: 16–17; FDA, Division of Dockets Management (Rockland, Md.). Obtained through Freedom of Information Act.

52. Arthur J. Prange et al., "Effects of Thyrotropin-Releasing Hormone in Depression," *Lancet*, 2 (Nov. 11, 1972): 999–1002. The authors noted, "Although our findings offer no direct evidence for hypothalamic underactivity in depression, such evidence exists" (p. 1001).

53. Arthur J. Prange, Jr., et al., "The Therapeutic Use of Hormones of the Thyroid Axis in Depression," in *Neurobiology of Mood Disorders*, ed. Robert M. Post and James C. Ballenger (Baltimore: Williams & Wilkins, 1984), 311–322; quote, 311.

54. Arthur J. Prange, Jr., "Psychoneuroendocrinology: A Commentary," *Psychiatric Clinics of North America*, 21 (1998): 491–505; quote, 498.

55. Ingrid Krog-Meyer et al., "Prediction of Relapse with the TRH Test and Prophylactic Amitriptyline in 39 Patients with Endogenous Depression," *AJP*, 141 (1984): 945–948.

56. Charles B. Nemeroff et al., "Neurotensin: Central Nervous System Effects of a Hypothalamic Peptide," *Brain Research*, 128 (1977): 485–496.

57. Franklin W[ayne] Furlong, "Thyrotropin-Releasing Hormone: Differential Antidepressant and Endocrinological Effects," *AJP*, 133 (1976): 1187–1190.

58. Arthur J. Prange, Jr., Charles B. Nemeroff, and Morris A. Lipton, "Behavioral Effects of Peptides: Basic and Clinical Studies," in *Psychopharmacology: A Generation of Progress*, ed. Morris A. Lipton, Alberto DiMascio and Keith F. Killam (New York: Raven, 1978), 441–458; quote, 450.

59. Martin P. Szuba et al., "Rapid Antidepressant Response After Nocturnal TRH Administration in Patients with Bipolar Type I and Bipolar Type II Major Depression," *Journal of Clinical Psychopharmacology*, 25 (2005): 325–330.

60. Peter T. Loosen and Arthur J. Prange, Jr., "Serum Thyrotropin Response to Thyrotropin-Releasing Hormone in Psychiatric Patients: A Review," *AJP*, 139 (1982): 405–416; quote, 405.

61. Alan B. Levy and Stephen L. Stern, "DST and TRH Stimulation Test in Mood Disorder Subtypes," *AJP*, 144 (1987): 472–475.

62. Bernard Carroll, personal communication to authors, Jan. 9, 2008.

63. Florian Holsboer, "Neuroendocrinology of Mood Disorders," in *Psychopharmacology: The Fourth Generation of Progress*, ed. Floyd E. Bloom and David J. Kupfer (New York: Raven Press, 1995), 957–969, see 964.

64. Mark S. Gold, A. L. Pottash, and Irl Extein, "Hypothyroidism and Depression: Evidence from Complete Thyroid Evaluation," *JAMA*, 245 (May 15, 1981): 1919–1922; quote, 1922.

65. Robert H. Howland, "Thyroid Dysfunction in Refractory Depression: Implications for Pathophysiology and Treatment," *Journal of Clinical Psychiatry*, 54 (1993): 47–54.

66. Holsboer, "Neuroendocrinology of Mood Disorders," 957–969; see esp. 964.

67. Prange, in *Triumph* (ed. Ban), 65.

68. Rex W. Cowdry, Thomas A. Wehr, Athanasios P. Zis, and Frederick K. Goodwin, "Thyroid Abnormalities Associated with Rapid-Cycling Bipolar Illness," *Archives of General Psychiatry*, 40 (1983): 414–420.

69. R[olf] Gjessing, "Disturbances of Somatic Functions in Catatonia with a Periodic Course, and Their Compensation," *Journal of Mental Science*, 84 (1938): 608–621.

70. Mark S. Bauer and Peter C. Whybrow, "Rapid Cycling Bipolar Affective Disorder, II: Treatment of Refractory Rapid Cycling with High-Dose Levothyroxine: A Preliminary Study," *Archives of General Psychiatry*, 47 (1990): 435–440.

71. R[ussell] T. Joffe, P. P. Roy-Byrne, Thomas W. Uhde, Robert M. Post, "Thyroid Function and Affective Illness: A Reappraisal," *Biological Psychiatry*, 19 (1984): 1685–1691; quote, 1687.

72. R[ussell] Joffe and W. Singer, "The Effect of Tricyclic Antidepressants on Basal Thyroid Hormone Levels in Depressed Patients," *Pharmacopsychiatry*, 23 (1990): 67–69; Richard C. Shelton, Sheilah Winn, Nosahare Ekhatore, and Peter T. Loosen, "The Effects of Antidepressants on the Thyroid Axis in Depression," *Biological Psychiatry*, 33 (1993): 120–126; quote, p. 124.

73. Bernard Carroll, personal communication, Oct. 21, 2008.

74. Russell Joffe, personal communication, Jan. 14, 2008.

75. Prange, "Psychoneuroendocrinology Commentary," 497.

76. Arthur Prange, personal communication, Jan. 13, 2008.

77. Robertas Bunevicius, Gintautas Kazanavicius, Rimas Zalinkevicius, and Arthur J. Prange, Jr., "Effects of Thyroxine as Compared with Thyroxine Plus Triiodothyronine in Patients with Hypothyroidism," *New England Journal of Medicine*, 340 (Feb. 11, 1999): 424–429.

78. Keith A. Gary et al., "The Thyrotropin-Releasing Hormone (TRH) Hypothesis of Homeostatic Regulation: Implications for TRH-Based Therapeutics," *Journal of Pharmacology and Experimental Therapeutics*, 305 (2003): 410–416.

79. Prange, in *Triumph* (ed. Ban), 65.

80. Samuel B. Guze, *Why Psychiatry Is a Branch of Medicine* (New York: Oxford University Press, 1992).

81. F[lorian] Holsboer et al., "Diagnostic Value of Dexamethasone Suppression Test in Depression," *Lancet*, 2 (Sept. 27, 1980): 706.

82. Bernard J. Carroll, "Dexamethasone Suppression Test in Depression," (letter), *Lancet*, 2 (Dec. 6, 1980): 1249.

83. F[lorian] Holsboer, "Repeated Dexamethasone Suppression Test during Depressive Illness: Normalisation of Test Result Compared with Clinical Improvement," *Journal of Affective Disorders*, 4 (1982): 93–101.

84. F[lorian] Holsboer et al., "Corticotropin-Releasing-Factor Induced Pituitary-Adrenal Response in Depression," (letter), *Lancet*, 1 (Jan. 7, 1984): 55.

85. F[lorian] Holsboer et al., "Blunted Corticotropin and Normal Cortisol Response to Human Corticotropin-Releasing Factor in Depression," (letter), *New England Journal of Medicine*, 311 (Oct. 25, 1984): 1127.

86. See, for example, Charles B. Nemeroff et al., "Elevated Concentrations of CSF Corticotropin-Releasing Factor-Like Immunoreactivity in Depressed Patients," *Science*, 226 (Dec. 14, 1984): 1342–1344; Stacey Heit, Michael J. Owens, Paul Plotsky, and Charles B. Nemeroff, "Corticotropin-Releasing Factor, Stress, and Depression," *The Neuroscientist*, 3 (1997): 186–194; L. Arborelius, M. J. Owens, P. M. Plotsky, and C[harles] B. Nemeroff, "The Role of Corticotropin-Releasing Factor in Depression and Anxiety Disorders," *Journal of Endocrinology*, 160 (1999): 1–12.

87. F[lorian] Holsboer, "The Rationale for Corticotropin-Releasing Hormone Receptor (CRH-R) Antagonists to Treat Depression and Anxiety," *Journal of Psychiatric Research*, 33 (1999): 181–214. The issue of whether CRH is elevated in depression has proven controversial. Carroll is a disbeliever: "The best evidence [of non-elevation] is from Philip Gold's group, who sampled CSF across 24 hours and documented low rather than elevated CSF CRH levels in hypercortisolemic melancholic depression. . . . In later studies of carefully diagnosed depressed suicides, there was no change in brain binding sites for CRH." (Carroll, personal communication to the authors, Jan. 9, 2008.) The Gold reference is Ma-Li Wong et al., "Pronounced and Sustained Central Hypernoradrenergic Function in Major Depression with Melancholic Features: Relation to Hypercortisolism and Corticotropin-Releasing Hormone," *Proceedings of the National Academy of Sciences*, 97 (Jan. 4, 2000): 325–330. The postmortem studies of cortisol in depressed suicide data are: David Hucks et al., "Corticotropin-Releasing Factor Binding Sites in Cortex of Depressed Suicides," *Psychopharmacology*, 134 (1997): 174–178; Alan Leake et al., "Cortical Concentrations of Corticotropin-Releasing Hormone and Its Receptor in Alzheimer-Type Dementia and Major Depression," *Biological Psychiatry*, 28 (1990): 603–608.

88. David Rubinow, interview with Edward Shorter and Max Fink, June 9, 2009, Chapel Hill, N.C.

89. Florian Holsboer, "Corticotropin-Releasing Hormone—A New Tool to Investigate Hypothalamic-Pituitary-Adrenocortical Physiology in Psychiatric Patients," *Psychopharmacology Bulletin*, 22 (1986): 907–912; quote, 909.

90. F[lorian] Holsboer et al., Stimulation Response to Corticotropin-Releasing Hormone (CRH) in Patients with Depression, Alcoholism and Panic Disorder," *Hormone and Metabolic Research*, suppl. 16 (1987): 80–88.

91. Ulrich von Bardeleben, Florian Holsboer, G. K. Stalla, and O. A. Müller, "Combined Administration of Human Corticotropin-Releasing Factor and Lysine Vasopressin Induces Cortisol Escape from Dexamethasone Suppression in Healthy Subjects," *Life Sciences*, 37 (1985): 1613–1618.

92. F[lorian] Holsboer et al., "Serial Assessment of Corticotropin-Releasing Hormone Response after Dexamethasone in Depression: Implications for Pathophysiology of DST Nonsuppression," *Biological Psychiatry*, 22 (1987): 228–234.

93. Ulrich von Bardeleben and Florian Holsboer, "Cortisol Response to a Combined Dexamethasone-Human Corticotrophin-Releasing Hormone Challenge in Patients with Depression," *Journal of Neuroendocrinology*, 1 (1989): 485–488.

94. U[lrich] von Bardeleben, K. Wiedemann, and F[lorian] Holsboer, "Kombinierter Corticotropin-Releasing-Hormone-Dexamethason-suppressionstest bei Patienten mit endogener Depression," in *Biologische Psychiatrie: Synopsis 1986/87*, ed. Helmut Beckmann and Gerd Laux (Berlin: Springer, 1988), 259–261.

95. Edith Holsboer-Trachsler, Rudolf Stohler, and Martin Hatzinger, "Repeated Administration of the Combined Dexamethasone-Human Corticotropin Releasing Hormone Stimulation Test During Treatment of Depression," *Psychiatry Research*, 38 (1991): 163–171.

96. Isabella Heuser, Alexander Yassourdis, and Florian Holsboer, "The Combined Dexamethasone/CRH Test: A Refined Laboratory Test for Psychiatric Disorders," *Journal of Psychiatry Research*, 28 (1994): 341–356.

97. Carroll, personal communication, Jan. 9, 2008.

98. Heuser, "Combined Dexamethasone/CRH Test," 341.

99. Angelika Ehrhardt et al., "Regulation of the Hypothalamic-Pituitary-Adrenocortical System in Patients with Panic Disorder," *Neuropsychopharmacology*, 31 (2006): 2515–2522; tables 4 and 5.

100. F[lorian] Holsboer, "The Rationale for Corticotropin-Releasing Hormone Receptor (CRH-R) Antagonists to Treat Depression and Anxiety," *Journal of Psychiatric Research*, 33 (1999): 181–214; see 181 et passim.

101. Bernard J. Carroll, George C. Curtis, and Joseph Mendels, "Neuroendocrine Regulation in Depression. I. Limbic System-Adrenocortical Dysfunction," *Archives of General Psychiatry*, 33 (1976): 1039–1044; quote, 1039.

102. Christine Heim et al., "The Dexamethasone/CRF Test in Men with Major Depression: Role of Childhood Trauma," in ACNP, Poster Session II, Dec. 13, 2005, *Neuropsychopharmacology*, 30 (2005): S173–S174.

103. Rubinow–Shorter/Fink interview, 2008.

104. Ibid.

105. Rainer Rupprecht et al., "Progesterone Receptor-Mediated Effects of Neuroactive Steroids," *Neuron*, 11 (1993): 523–530.

106. Elena Romeo et al., "Effects of Antidepressant Treatment on Neuroactive Steroids in Major Depression," *AJP*, 155 (1998): 910–913; quote, 910.

107. Bruce S. McEwen, J. M. Weiss, and L. S. Schwartz, "Selective Retention of Corticosterone by Limbic Structures in Rat Brain," *Nature*, 220 (Nov. 30, 1968): 911–912.

108. B[ernard] I. Grosser, W. Stevens, and D. J. Reed, "Properties of Corticosterone-Binding Macromolecules from Rat Brain Cytosol," *Brain Research*, 57 (1973): 387–395.

109. Hans-Rudolph Olpe and Bruce S. McEwen, "Glucocorticoid Binding to Receptor-Like Proteins in Rat Brain and Pituitary: Ontogenetic and Experimentally Induced Changes," *Brain Research*, 105 (1976): 121–128; quote, 126.

110. Florian Holsboer, "The Corticosteroid Receptor Hypothesis of Depression," *Neuropsychopharmacology*, 23 (2000): 477–501; quote, 477.

111. Conrad M. Swartz and Edward Shorter, *Psychotic Depression* (New York: Cambridge University Press, 2007).

112. Robert T. Rubin et al., "Selective Neuroendocrine Effects of Low-Dose Haloperidol in Normal Adult Men," *Psychopharmacology*, 47 (1976): 135–140.

113. Robert T. Rubin, "Career at the Interface of Neuroendocrinology, Psychopharmacology, and Psychiatry," in *Reflections* (ed. Ban), 564–567; quote, 565.

114. Anthony J. Rothschild et al., "The Dexamethasone Suppression Test as a Discriminator among Subtypes of Psychotic Patients," *BJP*, 141 (1982): 471–474; quote, 473.

115. Bernard J. Carroll, George C. Curtis, and J[oe] Mendels, "Cerebrospinal Fluid and Plasma Free Cortisol Concentrations in Depression," *Psychological Medicine*, 6 (1976): 235–244.

116. Anthony J. Rothschild et al., "Dexamethasone Increases Plasma Free Dopamine in Man," *Journal of Psychiatric Research*, 18 (1984): 217–223, quotes 217, 221.

117. Alan F. Schatzberg et al., "A Corticosteroid/Dopamine Hypothesis for Psychotic Depression and Related States," *Journal of Psychiatric Research*, 19 (1985): 57–64.

118. Alan F. Schatzberg and Anthony J. Rothschild, "The Roles of Glucocorticoid and Dopaminergic Systems in Delusional (Psychotic) Depression," *Annals of the New York Academy of Sciences*, 537 (1988): 462–471. In 2003 Rothschild claimed that in 1988 he and Schatzberg had discussed the use of drugs that block "cortisol receptor antagonists in the brain" (Anthony J. Rothschild, "The Hypothalamic-Pituitary-Adrenal Axis and Psychiatric Illness," in *Psychoneuroendocrinology: The Scientific Basis of Clinical Practice*, ed. Owen M. Wolkowitz and Rothschild [Washington, D.C.: American Psychiatric Pub, 2003], 139–163, see 152). But in 1988 they had merely pointed to this as a general strategy without naming drugs or supplying details.

119. See C. Lewis Ravaris et al., "Effect of Ketoconazole on a Hypophysectomized, Hypercortisolemic, Psychotically Depressed Woman," *Archives of General Psychiatry*, 45 (1988): 966–967.

120. Beverley E. P[earson] Murphy, "Some Studies of the Protein-Binding of Steroids and Their Application to the Routine Micro and Ultramicro Measurement of Various Steroids in Body Fluids by Competitive Protein-Binding Radioassay," *Journal of Clinical Endocrinology and Metabolism*, 27 (1967): 973–990. See also Murphy, "Application of the Property of Protein-Binding to the Assay of Minute Quantities of Hormones and Other Substances," *Nature*, 201 (Feb. 15, 1964): 679–682, where she raised the theoretical possibility.

121. Beverley Murphy, unpublished memoir, sent to authors Oct. 23, 2007.

122. Reported in Beverley E. Pearson Murphy, "Treatment of Major Depression with Steroid Suppressive Therapy," *Journal of Steroid Biochemistry and Molecular Biology*, 39 (1991): 239–244.

123. For the thoughts in this paragraph we are grateful to Bernard Carroll, personal communication, Jan. 9, 2008.

124. Beverley E. Pearson Murphy, "Steroids and Depression," *Journal of Steroid Biochemistry and Molecular Biology*, 38 (1991): 537–559; quotes, 554.

125. Beverley E. Pearson Murphy et al., "Response to Steroid Suppression in Major Depression Resistant to Antidepressant Therapy," *Journal of Clinical Psychopharmacology*, 11 (1991): 121–126.

126. Exchange of letters between Rothschild and Schatzberg, and Murphy, in *Journal of Clinical Psychopharmacology*, 12 (1992): 142–144.

127. See Lynette K. Nieman et al., "Successful Treatment of Cushing's Syndrome with the Glucocorticoid Antagonist RU 486," *Journal of Clinical Endocrinology and Metabolism*, 61 (1985): 536–540; Aart-Jan van der Lely, K. Foeken, A. C. van der Mast, and S. W. Lamberts, "Rapid Reversal of Acute Psychosis in the Cushing Syndrome with the Cortisol-Receptor Antagonist Mifepristone (RU 486)," *Annals of Internal Medicine*, 114 (1991): 143–144.

128. Beverley E. Pearson Murphy, Daniel Filippini, and A. Missagh Ghadirian, "Possible Use of Glucocorticoid Receptor Antagonists in the Treatment of Major Depression: Preliminary Results Using RU 486," *Journal of Psychiatry and Neuroscience*, 18 (1993): 209–213.

129. A. Missagh Ghadirian et al., "The Psychotropic Effects of Inhibitors of Steroid Biosynthesis in Depressed Patients Refractory to Treatment," *Biological Psychiatry*, 37 (1995): 369–375.

130. Beverley Murphy to Edward Shorter, Nov. 5, 2007.

131. Xavier Bertagna et al., "The New Steroid Analog RU 486 Inhibits Glucocorticoid Action in Man," *Journal of Clinical Endocrinology and Metabolism*, 59 (1984): 25–28; R. C. Gaillard et al., "RU 486: A Steroid with Antiglucocorticosteroid Activity That Only Disinhibits the Human Pituitary-Adrenal System at a Specific Time of Day," *Proceedings of the National Academy of Sciences*, 81, no. 12 (Part I; Biological Sciences) (June 15, 1984): 3879–3882. For an overview of this early research—which makes no reference to psychiatry—see Étienne-Émile Baulieu, "1993: RU 486—A Decade on Today and Tomorrow," in Institute of Medicine, *Clinical Applications of Mifepristone (RU 486) and Other Antiprogestins: Assessing the Science and Recommending a Research Agenda*, ed. Molla S. Donaldson, Laneta Dorflinger, Sarah S. Brown, and Leslie Z. Benet (Washington, D.C.: National Academy Press, 1993), 71–119.

132. Mitchell A. Kling et al., "Effects of Glucocorticoid Antagonism with RU 486 on Pituitary-Adrenal Function in Patients with Major Depression: Time-Dependent Enhancement of Plasma ACTH Secretion," *Psychopharmacology Bulletin*, 25 (1989): 466–472; quote, 472.

133. K. Ranga Rana Krishnan et al., "RU 486 in Depression," *Progress in Neuro-Psychopharmacology and Biological Psychiatry*, 16 (1992): 913–920; quote, 918.

134. See document marked "Mifepristone—Stanley," dated Feb. 20, 2001, in Bernard Carroll Papers, International Neuropsychopharmacology Archives, Eskind Biomedical Library, Vanderbilt University Medical Center, Nashville, Tenn.

135. Susan Freinkel, "The Case of the Notorious Depression Drug," *San Francisco Magazine*, May 2007: 56ff.

136. Charles DeBattista, Brent Solvason, Joseph Belanoff, and Alan F. Schatzberg, "Letter: Treatment of Psychotic Depression," *AJP*, 154 (1997): 1625–1626.

137. Anthony J. Rothschild, "Letter: Conflict-of-Interest Charge," *AJP*, 161 (2004): 1721–1722. Yet, one report stated that Rothschild did have a financial interest in Corcept. Joseph K. Belanoff et al., "An Open Label Trial of C-1073 (Mifepristone) for Psychotic Major Depression," *Biological Psychiatry*, 52 (2002): 386–392.

138. Alan Schatzberg, interview for the American College of Neuropsychopharmacology, Dec. 12, 2001; ACNP Video History Project; Collection Transcripts, interview #102, International Neuropsychopharmacology Archives, University of California, Los Angeles.

139. James W. Chu et al., "Successful Long-Term Treatment of Refractory Cushing's Disease with High-Dose Mifepristone (RU 486)," *Journal of Clinical Endocrinology and Metabolism*, 86 (2001): 3568–3573.

140. Joseph K. Belanoff et al., "Rapid Reversal of Psychotic Depression Using Mifepristone," *Journal of Clinical Psychopharmacology*, 21 (2001): 516–521.

141. Joseph K. Belanoff et al., "Cortisol and Cognitive Changes in Psychotic Major Depression," *AJP*, 158 (2001): 1612–1616.

142. See Belanoff, "Open-Label Trial."

143. Alan F. Schatzberg, "New Approaches to Managing Psychotic Depression," *Journal of Clinical Psychiatry*, 64, suppl. 1 (2003): 19–23; quote, 21.

144. Charles DeBattista et al., "Mifepristone versus Placebo in the Treatment of Psychosis in Patients with Psychotic Major Depression," *Biological Psychiatry*, 60 (2006): 1343–1349; the results were first reported at ACNP in 2004.

145. Robert T. Rubin and Bernard J. Carroll, "Claims for Mifepristone in Neuropsychiatric Disorders: Commentary on DeBattista and Belanoff, and Neigh and Nemeroff," *TRENDS in Endocrinology and Metabolism*, 17 (2006): 384–385; quote, 385; see also

Robert T. Rubin and Bernard J. Carroll, "Mifepristone (RU 486) in the Treatment of Psychotic Depression: Re-Evaluation of Published Data," ACNP 2004 Annual Meeting, Abstract No. 63, *Neuropsychopharmacology*, 29, suppl. 1 (2004): S203.

146. Benjamin H. Flores et al., "Clinical and Biological Effects of Mifepristone Treatment for Psychotic Depression," *Neuropsychopharmacology*, 31 (2006): 628–636. In fairness, an open-label trial of one week's duration (but patients followed for eight weeks) led by George Simpson at the University of Southern California, at two sites in Egypt, found some efficacy for mifepristone in depression up to four weeks (but not thereafter); the improvement in psychosis after four weeks was "of borderline significance." George M. Simpson, Adel El Sheshai, Nasser Loza, et al., "An 8-Week Open-Label Trial of a 6-Day Course of Mifepristone for the Treatment of Psychotic Depression," *Journal of Clinical Psychiatry*, 66 (2005), pp. 598–602.

147. Uriel Halbreich interview by Edward Shorter and Max Fink, Hollywood, Fla., Dec. 4, 2006.

148. Nandakumar Nagaraja et al., "Glucocorticoid Mechanisms May Contribute to ECT-Induced Retrograde Amnesia," *Psychopharmacology*, 190 (2007): 73–80.

149. Rubin and Carroll, "Mifepristone Re-Evaluation," who argue that Corcept had not made its case because its trials had not included measures of cortisol.

Notes to Chapter 8

1. U.S. Food and Drug Administration, Psychopharmacologic Drugs Advisory Committee, Transcript of meeting of Nov. 6, 1980 184; FDA, Division of Dockets Management (Rockland, Md.). Obtained through Freedom of Information Act.

2. Steven E. Hyman, "Can Neuroscience Be Integrated into the *DSM-V?*" *Nature Reviews/Neuroscience*, 8 (2007): 725–732; quote, 727.

3. Herman Van Praag, "Psychiatry and the March of Folly" (interview), in *The Psychopharmacologists*, [vol. 1], ed. David Healy (London: Altman, 1996), 353–379; quote, 367.

4. Frederick K. Goodwin and Kay Redfield Jamison, *Manic-Depressive Illness* (New York: Oxford University Press, 1990), 459. The second edition of their book in 2007, while discussing neuroendocrine findings extensively, contents itself with the blanket generalization, "While abnormalities in these multiple neurotransmitter and neuropeptide systems are involved in mood disorders, they likely represent the downstream effects of other, more primary abnormalities," meaning, as the authors go on to suggest, intracellular signaling changes. Goodwin and Jamison, *Manic-Depressive Illness: Bipolar Disorders and Recurrent Depression*, 2nd ed. (New York: Oxford University Press, 2007), 536.

5. *Neuropsychopharmacology: The Fifth Generation of Progress: An Official Publication of the American College of Neuropsychopharmacology*, ed. Kenneth L. Davis, Dennis Charney, Joseph T. Coyle, and Charles Nemeroff (Philadelphia: Lippincott, 2002).

6. Arthur Prange, personal communication to Edward Shorter, Nov. 2, 2007.

7. Paul McHugh interview with Max Fink, Dec. 10, 2007, Stony Brook, N.Y.

8. David Rubinow interview with Edward Shorter and Max Fink, June 9, 2008, Chapel Hill, N.C.

9. Marvin Stein, interview with Edward Shorter and Max Fink, Oct. 24, 2007.

10. McHugh–Fink interview, 2007.

11. We are anonymizing the name of this contributor to the listserv psycho-pharm@psycom.net, post of Feb. 13, 2008.

12. *Melancholia: A Disorder of Movement and Mood: A Phenomenological and Neurobiological Review*, ed. Gordon Parker and Dusan Hadzi-Pavlovic (Cambridge, U.K.: Cambridge University Press, 1996).

13. Michael Alan Taylor and Max Fink, *Melancholia: The Diagnosis, Pathophysiology, and Treatment of Depressive Illness* (Cambridge, U.K.: Cambridge University Press, 2006).

14. *Melancholia: Beyond DSM, Beyond Neurotransmitters*, ed. Tom G. Bolwig and Edward Shorter, *Acta Psychiatrica Scandinavica Supplementum*, 115, no. 433 (2007).

15. Walter Brown interview with Max Fink and Edward Shorter, Feb. 16, 2006, Tiverton, R.I.

Notes to Chapter 9

1. Max Fink, "Remembering the Lost Neuroscience of Pharmaco-EEG," *Acta Psychiatrica Scandinavica*, in press.

2. Max Fink, "Experimental Psychiatric Research at Hillside: Review and Prospect," *Journal of the Hillside Hospital*, 10 (1961): 159–169.

3. H. L. Rachlin et al., "Follow-up Studies of 317 Patients Discharged from Hillside Hospital in 1950," *Journal of the Hillside Hospital*, 5 (1956): 17–40.

4. Max Fink, Robert Shaw, George Gross, and Fred Coleman. "Comparative Study of Chlorpromazine and Insulin Coma in the Therapy of Psychosis," *JAMA*, 166 (1958): 1846–1850.

5. Max Fink, "*A Beautiful Mind* and Insulin Coma: Social Constraints on Psychiatric Diagnosis and Treatment," *Harvard Review of Psychiatry*, 11 (2003): 284–290. In retrospect, however, our conclusion was flawed because we did not separate the patients according to their illness; it is possible that the treatments had differential effects lost in the mixed samples. The sample size was also small, subjecting the conclusion to statistical error.

6. At the time, the new agents were prescribed by the research department clinicians, after referral by the patient's clinician. For details, see Fink, "Lost Neuroscience of Pharmaco-EEG," and Fink, "A Clinician-Researcher and ECDEU: 1959–1980," in *The Triumph of Psychopharmacology*, ed. Tom Ban, David Healy, and Edward Shorter (Budapest, Animula, 2000), 82–96.

7. Max Fink, Donald F. Klein, and John Kramer,"Clinical Efficacy of Chlorpromazine Procyclidine Combination, Imipramine and Placebo in Depressive Disorders," *Psychopharmacologia*, 7 (1965): 27–36.

8. Donald F. Klein and Max Fink, "Psychiatric Reaction Patterns to Imipramine," *AJP*, 119 (1962): 432–438.

9. Donald F. Klein and Max Fink, "Behavioral Reaction Patterns with Phenothiazines," *Archives of General Psychiatry*, 7 (1962): 449–459.

10. John Kramer, Donald Klein, and Max Fink. "Withdrawal Symptoms Following Discontinuation of Imipramine Therapy," *AJP*, 118 (1961): 549–550.

11. Richard Abrams and Michael A. Taylor, "A Comparison of Unipolar and Bipolar Depressive Illness," *AJP*, 137 (1980): 1084–1087.

12. Richard Abrams and Michael A. Taylor, "The Importance of Mood-Incongruent Psychotic Symptoms in Melancholia," *Journal of Affective Disorders*, 5 (1983): 179–181.

13. Michael A. Taylor and Richard Abrams, "The Phenomenology of Mania: A New Look at Some Old Patients," *Archives of General Psychiatry*, 29 (1973): 520–522.

14. Michael A. Taylor and Richard Abrams, "Reassessing the Bipolar-Unipolar Dichotomy," *Journal of Affective Disorders*, 2 (1980): 195–217.

15. Donald F. Klein, "The Pharmacological Validation of Psychiatric Diagnosis," in *The Validity of Psychiatric Diagnosis*, ed. Lee N. Robins and James E. Barrett (New York: Raven Press, 1989), 177–201.

16. Max Fink and Michael A. Taylor, *Catatonia: A Clinician's Guide to Diagnosis and Treatment* (Cambridge, U.K.: Cambridge University Press, 2003).

17. Michael A. Taylor and Max Fink, "Catatonia in Psychiatric Classification: A Home of Its Own," *AJP*, 160 (2003): 1233–1241.

18. Michael A. Taylor and Max Fink, *Melancholia: The Diagnosis, Pathophysiology and Treatment of Depressive Illness* (Cambridge, U.K.: Cambridge University Press, 2006).

19. Michael A. Taylor and Max Fink, "Restoring Melancholia in the Classification of Mood Disorders," *Journal of Affective Disorders*, 105 (2008): 1–14.

20. Max Fink and Michael A. Taylor, "The Medical Evidence-Based Model to Identify Psychiatric Syndromes: Return to a Classical Paradigm," *Acta Psychiatrica Scandinavica*, 87 (2008): 81–84.

21. *Hormones, Behavior and Psychopathology*, ed. Edward J. Sachar (New York: Raven Press, 1976).

22. Bernard J. Carroll, George C. Curtis, and Joseph Mendels, "Neuroendocrine Regulation in Depression. II: Discrimination of Depressed from Nondepressed Patients," *Archives of General Psychiatry*, 33 (1976): 1051–1057.

23. *Depressive Illness: Some Research Studies*, ed. Brian Davies, Bernard J. Carroll, and Robert M. Mowbray (Springfield, Ill.: C.C. Thomas, 1972).

24. Peter T. Loosen and Arthur Prange, "Thyrotropin Releasing Hormone (TRH): A Useful Tool for Psychoendocrine Investigation," *Psychoneuroendocrinology*, 5 (1980): 63–80.

25. Yiannis Papakostas et al., "Neuroendocrine Measures in Psychiatric Patients: Course and Outcome with ECT," *Psychiatry Research*, 4 (1981): 55–64.

26. Max Fink, *Electroshock: Restoring the Mind* (New York: Oxford University Press, 1999).

27. *Psychobiology of Convulsive Therapy*, ed. Max Fink, Seymour Kety, and James McGaugh (Washington, D.C.: V.H. Winston & Sons, 1974.)

28. Unpublished transcript, dated April 21, 1978, of the meeting sponsored by the National Institute of Mental Health held February 22–24, 1978, in New Orleans, Max Fink Collection, Special Collections, Stony Brook University Libraries, Stony Brook, N.Y. A few years earlier Abrams and Taylor had also called attention to the role of the diencephalon in ECT. Richard Abrams and Michael Alan Taylor, "Diencephalic Stimulation and the Effects of ECT in Endogenous Depression," *British Journal of Psychiatry*, 129 (1976): 482–485.

29. Jan-Otto Ottosson, *Experimental Studies of the Mode of Action of Electroconvulsive Therapy* (Copenhagen: Ejnar Munksgaard, 1960).

30. Martin Roth, "Changes in EEG under Barbiturate Anesthesia Produced by Electro-convulsive Treatment and Their Significance for a Theory of ECT Action," *Electroencephalography and Clinical Neurophysiology*, 3 (1951): 261–280.

31. Max Fink, *Convulsive Therapy: Theory and Practice* (New York: Raven Press, 1979).

32. Max Fink and Jan-Otto Ottosson. "A Theory of Convulsive Therapy in Endogenous Depression: Significance of Hypothalamic Dysfunction," *Psychiatry Research*, 2 (1980): 49–61.

33. Alexander H. Glassman, Shepard J. Kantor, and Michael Shostak, "Depression, Delusions and Drug Response," *AJP*, 132 (1975): 716–719.

34. David Avery and A. Lubrano, "Depression Treated with Imipramine and ECT: The DeCarolis Study Reconsidered," *AJP*, 136 (1979): 559–562.

35. Duane G. Spiker, James Stein, and Charles Rich, "Delusional Depression and Electroconvulsive Therapy: One Year Later," *Convulsive Therapy*, 1 (1985) 167–172. (We now know that almost all psychotic depressed patients are melancholic.)

36. Taylor and Fink, *Melancholia*.

37. Joseph Schildkraut, S. Schanberg, George Breese, and Irwin Kopin. "Norepinephrine Metabolism and Drugs Used in Affective Disorders: A Possible Mechanism of Action," *AJP*, 124 (1967): 600–608.

38. Charles Nemeroff, Garth Bissette, Huda Akil, and Max Fink, "Neuropeptide Concentrations in the Cerebrospinal Fluid of Depressed Patients Treated with Electroconvulsive Therapy: Corticotrophin-Releasing Factor, Beta-Endorphin and Somatostatin," *British Journal of Psychiatry*, 158 (1991): 59–63.

39. Robert Keisling, "Successful Treatment of an Unidentified Patient with One ECT," *AJP*, 141 (1984): 148. Charles Rich, "Recovery from Depression After One ECT," *AJP*, 141 (1984): 1010–1011.

40. Max Fink "How Does Convulsive Therapy Work?" *Neuropsychopharmacology*, 3 (1990): 730–782; Max Fink "Response to Critiques," ibid., 97–100.

41. Max Fink and Michael A. Taylor, "Electroconvulsive Therapy: Evidence and Challenges," *JAMA*, 298 (2007): 330–332.

42. Charles H. Kellner et al. "Continuation ECT vs. Pharmacotherapy for Relapse Prevention in Major Depression: A Multisite Study from the Consortium for Research in Electroconvulsive Therapy (CORE)," *Archives of General Psychiatry*, 63 (2006):1337–1344; Georgios Petrides et al., "ECT Remission Rates in Psychotic Versus Nonpsychotic Depressed Patients: A Report from CORE." *Journal of ECT*, (2001) 17: 244–253.

43. Personal records of research grant applications, Max Fink Collection, Special Collections, Stony Brook University Libraries, Stony Brook, N.Y.

44. Max Fink, *Electroshock: Restoring the Mind* (New York: Oxford University Press, 1999).

45. Max Fink, "Electroshock Revisited," *American Scientist*, 88 (2000): 162–167.

46. Jan-Otto Ottosson and Max Fink, *Ethics in Electroconvulsive Therapy* (New York: Brunner-Routledge, 2004).

47. Gregory L. Fricchione, L. D. Kaufman, B. L. Gruber, and Max Fink, "Electroconvulsive Therapy and Cyclophosphamide in Combination for Severe Neuropsychiatric Lupus with Catatonia," *American Journal of Medicine*, 88 (1990): 443–444.

48. Fink and Taylor, *Catatonia*.

49. B. Mahendra, "Where Have All the Catatonics Gone?" *Psychological Medicine*, 11 (1981): 669–671.

50. Max Fink, "Catatonia. A Syndrome Appears, Disappears, and Is Rediscovered," *Canadian Journal of Psychiatry*, 54 (2009): 23–31.

51. George Bush et al., "Catatonia: I: Rating Scale and Standardized Examination," *Acta Psychiatrica Scandinavica*, 93 (1996): 129–136; Bush, "Catatonia: II: Treatment with Lorazepam and Electroconvulsive Therapy," ibid., 137–143.

52. J. R. Morrison, "Catatonia: Diagnosis and Treatment," *Hospital and Community Psychiatry*, 26 (1975): 91–94; Richard Abrams and Michael Alan Taylor, "Catatonia, a Prospective Clinical Study," *Archives of General Psychiatry*, 33 (1976): 579–581.

53. Max Fink and Michael A. Taylor, "Catatonia: A Separate Category for DSM-IV?" *Integrative Psychiatry*, 7 (1991): 2–10.

54. American Psychiatric Association, *Diagnostic and Statistical Manual of Mental Disorders*, *Fourth Edition.* (Washington, D.C.: APA 1994).

55. Taylor and Fink, "Catatonia: A Home of Its Own."
56. Max Fink and Michael A. Taylor, "Catatonia: Subtype or Syndrome in *DSM?*" *AJP*, 163 (2006): 1875–1876.
57. Fink and Taylor, *Catatonia*.
58. William J. Bleckwenn, "Catatonia Cases After IV Sodium Amytal Injection" (Videotape, 1930); Washington, D.C.: National Library of Medicine. NLM ID:8501040A (visual material).
59. Laszlo Meduna, *Die Konvulsionstherapie der Schizophrenie* (Halle, Germany: Carl Marhold Verlagsbuchhandlung, 1937); Gábor Gazdag et al., "László Meduna's Pilot Studies with Camphor Inductions of Seizures: The First 11 Patients," *Journal of ECT*, 25 (2009): 3–11.
60. Bush, "Catatonia: II."
61. Max Fink and Michael A. Taylor. "The Many Varieties of Catatonia," *European Archives of Psychiatry and Clinical Neuroscience*, 251 (2001), Suppl. I: I8–I13.
62. Fink and Taylor, *Catatonia: From Psychopathology to Neurobiology*, ed. Stanley N. Caroff et al. (Washington, D.C.: American Psychiatric Press, 2004).
63. Dirk M. Dhosshe, Lorna Wing, Masataka Ohta, and Klaus-Jürgen Neumärker, "Catatonia in Autism Spectrum Disorders," *International Review of Biology 72* (Amsterdam: Academic Press, 2006); Lee E. Wachtel et al., "ECT for Catatonia in an Autistic Girl," *AJP*, 165 (2008): 329–333.
64. Max Fink, *Electroshock: Healing Mental Illness* (New York: Oxford University Press, 1999).
65. Gino Pozzi et al., "Is Catatonia a Separate Entity Related to Affective Disorders?" *European Journal of Psychiatry*, 12 (1998): 32–44.
66. Taylor and Fink, *Melancholia*.
67. Davies, *Depressive Illness*.
68. Max Fink, "Should the Dexamethasone Suppression Test Be Resurrected?" *Acta Psychiatrica Scandinavica*, 112 (2005): 245–249.
69. A. John Rush, "STAR*D: What Have We Learned?" *AJP*, 164 (2007): 201–204; A. John Rush et al., "Acute and Longer-Term Outcomes in Depressed Outpatients Requiring One or Several Treatment Steps: A STAR*D Report," *AJP*, 163 (2006): 1905–1917.
70. Chapter 6, this volume.
71. Eli Robins and Samuel Guze, "Establishment of Diagnostic Validity in Psychiatric Illness, Its Application to Schizophrenia," *AJP*, 126 (1970): 983–987.
72. Edward Shorter, *Before Prozac* (New York: Oxford University Press, 2009).

Index